Contemporary
and Management of
Heart
Failure®

Barry H. Greenberg, MD
Professor of Medicine
Director, Heart Failure/
Cardiac Transplantation Program
University of California-San Diego

Denise D. Hermann, MD
Assistant Director, Heart Failure/
Cardiac Transplantation Program
University of California-San Diego

First Edition

Published by
Handbooks in Health Care Co.,
Newtown, Pennsylvania, USA

International Standard Book Number: 98-74009

Library of Congress Catalog Card Number: 1-884065-46-5

Contents

This book has been prepared and is presented as a service to the medical community. The information provided reflects the knowledge, experience, and personal opinions of Barry H. Greenberg, MD, Professor of Medicine, and Director, Heart Failure/Cardiac Transplantation Program, and Denise D. Hermann, MD, Assistant Director, Heart Failure/Cardiac Transplantation Program, University of California, San Diego, CA.

This book is not intended to replace or to be used as a substitute for the complete prescribing information prepared by each manufacturer for each drug. Because of possible variations in drug indications, in dosage information, in newly described toxicities, in drug/drug interactions, and in other items of importance, reference to such complete prescribing information is definitely recommended before any of the drugs discussed are used or prescribed.

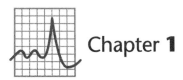

Chapter **1**

Pathophysiology of Heart Failure

eart failure has been recognized as a clinical syndrome since the ancient Egyptian and early Greek civilizations. However, despite our long-standing ability to identify the signs and symptoms of heart failure, the definitions used to describe this syndrome have evolved substantially over time. This progressive redefinition of heart failure is based on input from several sources. New insights have been made on the basis of observations made by astute clinicians, and results of clinical trials assessing new therapies have also helped support (or refute) various ideas about the causes of heart failure. The clinical database has been complemented and often stimulated by mechanistic and therapeutic studies in experimental animal models and by basic laboratory work that has unraveled many of the cellular processes and pathways that lie at the roots of this syndrome. Most recently, our understanding of the basis of heart failure has been extended by insights gained using the techniques of molecular biology and by the pioneering work of defining the human genome.

The continued evolution of our understanding of heart failure pathophysiology has resulted in a succession of paradigms to describe this syndrome. Figure 1 depicts the paradigms that have been used over the past 50 years. These paradigms help us clinically because they provide

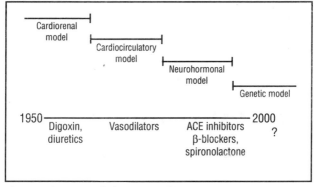

Figure 1: Heart failure paradigms.

a rationale for many of the therapies that are currently being used or evaluated for the treatment of heart failure. However, in reality, no single paradigm suffices as a complete description of heart failure because each one listed in Figure 1 describes only an aspect of the syndrome. All are correct, but none are by themselves sufficient. Thus, depending on the purpose, a clinician might use one or more of these paradigms to help explain a particular clinical or mechanistic aspect of heart failure. As we shall see, however, the neurohormonal model of heart failure that has been developed over the past 20 years dominates our thinking about heart failure pathophysiology and has provided a basis for many of the new and highly effective therapies that have emerged for the treatment of heart failure.

For the purposes of the clinician, a useful definition is one proposed by Philip Poole-Wilson in 1985, in which he defined heart failure as "a clinical syndrome caused by an abnormality of the heart and recognized by a characteristic pattern of haemodynamic, renal, neural and hormonal responses." This definition incorporates many aspects of the cardiorenal, cardiocirculatory, and neurohormonal paradigms depicted in Figure 1 and could be further extended by adding that when heart failure develops, the heart is unable to provide adequate amounts of oxygenated blood to meet the needs of peripheral tissue or is able to do so only at abnormally high intracardiac filling pressures. This addition incorporates many of the signs and symptoms of heart failure that appear in our patients.

It is worth pointing out that the term *heart failure* rather than *congestive heart failure* is used in this definition and throughout this handbook in recognition of the fact that many patients with heart failure may not have evidence of congestion. For example, a patient with acutely decompensated heart failure caused by severely depressed left ventricular (LV) systolic function is admitted to the hospital with pulmonary edema and is subsequently diuresed, so that signs and symptoms of volume overload are abolished. In this case, many of the abnormalities in cardiac structure and function, circulatory hemodynamics, and neurohormonal activation persist despite the resolution of congestive signs and symptoms. The issue is more than merely a semantic one, since many physicians might be tempted to consider this patient to be free of heart failure (and at low risk for future events) once problems with fluid overload have been adequately treated. This approach, however, fails to recognize that the underlying progression of cardiac dysfunction caused by remodeling of the heart will continue and that this patient remains at high risk for future morbidity and mortality despite adequate treatment of the signs and symptoms of congestion.

Heart failure is a syndrome that can be caused by a variety of conditions that result in damage to the myocardium. These include such diverse conditions as myocardial infarction (MI), long-standing pressure or volume overload, myocyte damage caused by a viral infection, and damage caused by replacement of normal myocardium by infiltrative diseases, such as amyloidosis. Regardless of the cause, however, both the systemic response to altered cardiac function and the structural changes (and cellular processes) that develop within the heart itself in response to the initial injury are remarkably consistent. Thus, a characteristic of heart failure is that damage to the heart or prolonged increases in loading conditions result in a prototypic systemic and local cardiac neurohormonal response. The long-term effects of this widespread neurohormonal activation include changes in the structure and function of heart cells that were not initially damaged. This extension of the condition throughout the heart explains the progressive nature of the deterioration in cardiac function that occurs in heart failure patients. Although many of these structural and cellular changes were believed to be irreversible, there is now good evidence that both medical therapy and mechanical unloading of the heart can result in considerable recovery of cardiac function and reversion of the heart itself to a more normal structure. Thus, contemporary therapy of heart failure not only reduces morbidity and mortality, but also favorably affects the underlying processes that cause heart failure to progress. Recognition of this aspect of current therapy is central to the optimal prescription of therapies for heart failure patients.

Abnormalities in Cardiac Function

The diagnosis of heart failure on the basis of systolic dysfunction implies an abnormality in the pumping capacity of the heart. If mechanical problems (ie, with cardiac filling or emptying [caused by valvular or pericardial disease] or movement of blood within the heart [on the basis of intracardiac shunting]) are excluded, the basis of this abnormality resides in an inability of the myocardium to generate adequate amounts of force with each contraction. Thus, heart failure is characterized by abnormal shortening of individual sarcomeres, which may be further worsened by abnormalities in the interstitium or extracellular matrix (ECM) of the heart. Conditions that can result in abnormal cardiac sarcomere shortening are summarized in Table 1, which is based on an excellent recent review of the subject by Braunwald and Bristow.

Table 1: Basis of Cardiac Failure

Abnormalities in energy metabolism
- Relative subendocardial myocardial ischemia
- Reduced high-energy (eg, creatine phosphate [CRP]) stores
- Mitochondrial abnormalities
- Reduced creatine kinase activity

Alteration in expression or activity of contractile proteins (ie, reversion to the 'fetal gene pattern')
- Alterations in myosin heavy chain (MHC), troponin T, and myosin light chain-I

Abnormalities in excitation-contraction coupling
- Prolongation of intracellular Ca^+ transient
- Increased diastolic Ca^+ concentrations

Cytoskeletal abnormalities
- Excessive microtubular polymerization
- Increased cytoskeletal proteins (eg, tubulin, dystrophin)
- Decreased cytoskeletal proteins (eg, α-actinin, titin)
- Cytoskeletal gene mutations in dystrophin, desmin, sarcoglycans, and laminin A and C

Alterations in β-adrenergic signaling

An abnormality in energy metabolism refers to an inability of the heart to generate adequate energy within the myocytes, resulting in compromised shortening of the contractile units (sarcomeres). This may result from a variety of causes, including the effects of myocardial ischemia, presence of hypertrophy, reduction of high-energy creatine phosphate stores in the failing heart, mitochondrial abnormalities, and reduced activity of critical enzymes, such as creatine kinase. In all of these cases, the external work performed by the heart is compromised, while energy consumption remains in the normal or nearly normal range. Thus, the efficiency of cardiac function in the failing heart is abnormal.

In the setting of heart failure, evidence shows that the pattern of expression of several genes within the heart is altered. Most commonly, the changes in gene expression seen in the failing heart seem to recapitulate the pattern seen during early development of the organism. This transition involves both quantitative changes in gene expression and changes in the expressed isoform of genes encoding important structural and functional proteins in the heart. The changes in gene expression in the failing heart have been termed a *reversion to the fetal gene pattern* because many of the changes are similar to those seen during early development. Changes in gene expression that result in differences in cardiac contractile proteins have been described in both experimental animal models and human patients with heart failure. Examples include alterations in the expression of isoforms of myosin heavy chain (MHC), of the regulatory protein troponin T, and in the isoform expression of myosin light chain-I.

Abnormalities in excitation-contraction coupling have also been identified in the failing heart. In the end-stage failing human heart, prolongation of the calcium transient and increased diastolic calcium concentrations have been reported. These abnormalities are associated with the altered expression of genes for molecules such as sarcoplasmic reticular ATPase (SERCA) and its regulatory protein, phospholamban, both of which play an important role in the regulation of intracellular calcium concentrations. Abnormally low expression of the trans-sarcolemmal Na^+/Ca^{2+} transporter, which helps remove calcium from the myocyte, has also been reported in heart failure and may result in similar effects on intracellular calcium fluxes.

The cytoskeleton of cardiac myocytes is involved in the efficient transduction of sarcomere shortening to shortening and force generation within the cell. A variety of cytoskeletal proteins, such as dystrophin, laminin, actinin, titin, and myomesin, play a role in this process, and several mutations in cytoskeletal genes have been shown to be involved in the pathogenesis of dilated cardiomyopathy in human patients. Acquired abnormalities in the cytoskeleton have also been demonstrated in experimental models of heart failure. For example, pressure overload results in excessive microtubular polymerization that adversely affects the systolic function of the heart, and there is evidence that viral infection may adversely affect cardiac function through alterations in the cytoskeleton.

In addition, there is evidence that alterations in β-adrenergic receptor signal transduction play an important role in the pathogenesis of heart failure. Multiple signaling abnormalities have been implicated in this process, including down-regulation of the β_1-adrenergic receptor on cardiac myocytes. The net effect is reduction in cardiac reserve and impairment of exercise capacity in heart failure patients.

Compensatory Mechanisms

The compensatory mechanisms that develop in the setting of heart failure are outlined in Table 2. Generally, they are activated as a means of compensating for a reduction in arterial perfusion pressure. They are usually best suited to providing short-term support for the cardiovascular system during periods of acute stress, since they serve the useful purpose of augmenting cardiac output and maintaining arterial pressure.

It is tempting to consider that these mechanisms may have developed during evolution as means of protection from decreased perfusion pressure caused by dehydration and blood loss. However, the sustained activation of these compensatory mechanisms in response to diminished cardiac output or arterial perfusion pressure caused by car-

Table 2: Compensatory Mechanisms to Support the Failing Heart

Mechanism	Beneficial Effect
Immediate	
Salt/water retention	Increased intravascular volume resulting in increased CO and BP
Peripheral vasoconstriction	Increased venous return to the heart and augmented BP
Increased heart rate	Increased CO
Increased myocardial contractility	Increased CO
Long-term	
Myocardial hypertrophy	Increased force generation caused by an increased number of contractile units (ie, sarcomeres) Normalization of the wall stress
Chamber dilation	Increased stroke volume

BP = blood pressure
CO = cardiac output

diac dysfunction is now recognized to have long-term consequences that are mostly deleterious. An example of this is the retention of salt and water that develops in response to a reduction in cardiac output and arterial perfusion pressure. Initially, this results in an expansion of intracardiac volumes, which serves to increase cardiac output. However, this volume expansion also leads to worsening signs and symptoms of congestion and to an

Deleterious Consequence

Increased wall stress
Pulmonary and systemic congestion

Increased wall stress
Pulmonary congestion

Increased myocardial oxygen consumption

Increased myocardial oxygen consumption

Abnormalities in structural and functional
proteins within the myocyte
Energy supply/demand mismatch
Increased fibrosis

Increased wall stress
2° valvular insufficiency

increased load on the heart. The resultant increase in wall
stress, as we shall see later in this chapter, promotes adverse changes in cardiac structure that result in progressive deterioration in cardiac function.

Cardiac Remodeling

In response to myocardial injury or to prolonged increases in pressure and/or volume load, the heart under-

Table 3: Characteristics of Cardiac Remodeling

1. Initiated by damage to the heart, such as myocardial injury or increased pressure or volume load

2. Often continues even after resolution of initiating event

3. Tends to progress over time

4. Results in increased cardiac chamber volumes and muscle mass (eccentric hypertrophy), as well as increased ECM deposition

goes a prototypic series of changes in structure now commonly referred to as *cardiac remodeling*. In this process, eccentric hypertrophy of the myocardium develops, so there is an increase in both muscle mass and chamber volume of the left ventricle. Increased deposition of fibrous tissue in the ECM and alterations in the collagen characteristics also occur. The net effect of these changes is a progressive deterioration in both systolic and diastolic function of the heart. Characteristics of the remodeling process are summarized in Table 3. It is important to recognize that cardiac remodeling often continues well after the initiating event has resolved. Thus, even in the absence of continued or repetitive insults to the heart, remodeling may progress in an insidious manner, accounting for the all-too-common occurrence of heart failure as the first indication of a long-standing process that has resulted in extensive cardiac dysfunction.

The process of cardiac remodeling has been recognized in the post-MI population for some time, and most of our understanding of the clinical characteristics of cardiac remodeling comes from this population. For many years, researchers have known that patients who experience large MIs or who have substantial amounts of myocardial damage because of repeated episodes of injury are at high risk for cardiac remodeling. Initially, remodeling involves primarily the infarct zone, in which necrotic myocardium is replaced by scar tissue. However, even during this early phase, there is evidence that structural changes also occur in the noninfarcted segments of the heart. Activation of matrix metalloproteinases (MMPs), a family of proteolytic enzymes, occurs and results in ventricular dilatation caused by breakdown of the ECM of the heart. Later, further dilatation and hypertrophy of these noninfarcted segments occur so that what started as a discrete area of injury caused by an infarction progresses to a global process involving virtually all segments of the left ventricle.

The impact of remodeling on the clinical course is substantial. Increases in ventricular volumes are associated with an increased risk of future cardiac events, including onset of heart failure, hospitalization, and death. Whereas hypertrophy was once considered a beneficial compensatory response, the adverse consequences of hypertrophy in the remodeling heart have now become apparent. A study of patients in the Studies of Left Ventricular Dysfunction (SOLVD) trials and registry followed the clinical course of patients with heart failure over a 12-month period. Patients with an LV mass above the median value for the group had nearly a twofold increase in the likelihood of experiencing a cardiovascular event compared to patients whose mass was below the median value. Interestingly, the effect of increased mass on risk of future events was independent of the level of LV ejection fraction (EF). Patients with a myocardial mass above the median value for the group continued to be at a greater risk for mortality or cardiovascular hospitalization regardless of whether their EF was above or below 0.35. These findings implicate increases in myocardial mass as a negative prognostic factor in heart failure with either preserved or abnormal LV systolic function.

Although the connections between cardiac remodeling and abnormalities in contractile dysfunction are complex, the mechanisms involved are beginning to be elucidated. Many of the pathways activated in the course of the development of cardiac hypertrophy also play a role in the development of myocardial dysfunction. These include abnormalities in calcium handling, abnormal myocardial energetics, and induction of the fetal gene program. Increased amounts of ECM are also found in the remodeled hypertrophic heart and appear to play a particularly important role in patients with advanced systolic dysfunction. In a study of end-stage human ischemic cardiomyopathy, Beltrami et al noted that approximately two thirds of the fibrous tissue found in the remodeling heart was located outside of the regions of previous MI. Since fibrosis can impair both systolic and diastolic function of the heart, it seems likely that excess deposition of ECM in the remodeling heart is an important contributor to the progression of heart failure in this group.

During remodeling, increases in myocardial mass and chamber size are accompanied by changes in the heart configuration. The normal left ventricle is ellipsoid in shape. As the remodeling process progresses, this chamber takes on a more spherical shape. These increases in volume and mass and changes in the shape of the heart adversely affect the efficiency of contraction. As a result of dilatation of the valve annulus and abnormalities in the orientation of the various components of the subvalvular apparatus, remodeling also predisposes patients to secondary mitral and tricuspid valvular regurgitation. Thus, as the remodeling process continues and contractility begins to deteriorate, pump efficiency is also impaired by the development of tricuspid and mitral regurgitation. In this way, the structural changes that were initiated as a means of bolstering the failing heart ultimately lead to progressive worsening in cardiac performance.

Myocyte Apoptosis

As the heart remodels, there is evidence that a progressive loss of cardiac myocytes over time contributes to de-

Table 4: Characteristics of Apoptosis

1. Active, precisely regulated, energy-requiring process

2. Orchestrated by a genetic program

3. Plays a crucial role in regulating proliferating cell populations in adult tissues and in normal tissue development

Adapted from Sabbah HN: Apoptotic cell death in heart failure. *Cardiovasc Res* 2000;45:704-712.

terioration in cardiac function. While myocyte death caused by myocardial ischemia and toxic effects of neurohormonal agents, such as norepinephrine and angiotensin II (Ang II), appears to be involved in this process, there is evidence that myocyte loss caused by other factors may also play a role. Specifically, a growing body of evidence from experimental animal models and from human patients suggests that cardiac cell death caused by apoptosis occurs after MI and as LV dysfunction progresses. Apoptosis is an active process about which a great deal has been learned over the past decade. Some of the important characteristics of this type of programmed cell death are summarized in Table 4.

The causes of myocyte apoptosis in the heart appear to be diverse. Factors that can trigger apoptosis have been identified in various experimental animal models and in cell culture experiments; some of the most important ones are listed in Table 5. Evidence of apoptosis has been obtained in human hearts from patients with ischemic as well as nonischemic cardiomyopathies. Researchers estimate that apoptosis may result in the loss of 1% to 5% of cardiomyocytes each year in the failing human heart, a figure that, if correct, may well explain many aspects of the progressive nature of heart failure. Future heart failure therapies may

Table 5: Causes of Cardiomyocyte Apoptosis

1. Free oxygen radicals
2. Angiotensin II
3. Hypoxia
4. Cytokines (ie, TNF-α)
5. Calcium overload
6. Norepinephrine

be directed toward trying to block further worsening in cardiac function by inhibiting myocyte apoptosis. However, this issue is complicated by the fact that apoptosis is an important protective mechanism to help control unrestricted cell growth, and systemic blockade of this process would likely result in an increased risk of malignancies.

Causes of Cardiac Remodeling

Much work has been carried out over the years in identifying the causes of cardiac remodeling. The major factors involved in the pathogenesis of remodeling are outlined in Table 6. The effects of either pressure load or volume load in causing structural changes in the heart have been recognized for some time. Both situations result in an increase in wall stress. However, although both initiate remodeling, the pattern that develops is somewhat different in each instance.

Pressure overload, such as occurs with hypertension or aortic stenosis, results in the development of concentric hypertrophy. In contrast, volume overload that occurs with conditions such as aortic or mitral regurgitation produces eccentric hypertrophy of the left ventricle. Although there is an increase in muscle mass in each of these types of hypertrophy, dilatation of the ventricle accompanies volume overload but not pressure overload. In pure pressure over-

Table 6: Causes of Cardiac Remodeling

Hemodynamic Factors
- Pressure overload
- Volume overload

Neurohormonal Factors
- Angiotensin II
- Catecholamines
- Cytokines such as TNF-α
- Endothelin

load, the size of the ventricle does not increase at least until systolic dysfunction develops and the ventricle begins to fail. The remodeling that accompanies either pressure or volume overload is very much a compensatory response that enables the heart to accommodate changes in loading conditions and still maintain relatively normal function for an extended period. However, if the stimulus for continued growth and remodeling persists, cardiac function begins to deteriorate and heart failure ensues. The reasons for this are related to changes in cardiac cell phenotype that develop in the hypertrophic heart; myocardial oxygen supply-demand mismatches; and the adverse consequences of increased deposition of ECM within the heart. As noted previously, the presence of increased myocardial mass in heart failure patients with either preserved or impaired LV systolic function is an important negative prognostic risk factor.

Neurohormonal agents play a critical role in the remodeling process. Although many neurohormonal systems are activated during the development of heart failure, the effects of Ang II, norepinephrine (NE), endothelin (ET), and proinflammatory cytokines (such as tumor necrosis factor-α [TNF-α]) appear to have the most important effects on the remodeling process (Table 7). The central position

Table 7: Effects of Neurohormonal Agents on Cardiac Remodeling

Agent	Effect on Cardiac Load
Ang II	Increases salt/water retention Increases peripheral resistance
NE	Increases salt/water retention Increases peripheral resistance
ET	Increases salt/water retention
TNF-α	

Ang II = angiotensin II
ECM = extracellular matrix
ET = endothelin
MMPs = matrix metalloproteinases

of neurohormonal activation in the pathogenesis of heart failure is outlined in Figure 2.

Generally, the effects of the various neurohormonal agents activated in the failing heart tend to work in a synergistic

Effect on Cardiac Cells/ECM

Stimulates myocyte hypertrophy
Stimulates fibroblasts to produce ECM
Increases production of TIMPs that block ECM breakdown

Stimulates myocyte hypertrophy
Stimulates fibroblasts to produce ECM

Stimulates myocyte hypertrophy
Stimulates fibroblasts to produce ECM

Stimulates myocyte hypertrophy
Activates MMPs that break down ECM
Depresses myocardial contractility

Effect on Other Neurohormonal Systems

Stimulates prejunctional receptors on adrenergic nerves to release NE
Stimulates cardiac cells to release ET

Stimulates release of renin activity from the kidney

NE = norepinephrine
TIMPs = tissue inhibitors of metalloproteinases
TNF = tumor necrosis factor

fashion to initiate the compensatory changes outlined earlier in the chapter. The early effects of neurohormonal activation, such as salt and water retention and peripheral vasoconstriction, tend to increase both the pressure and

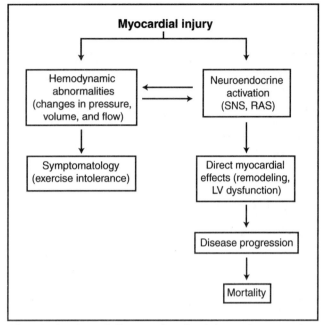

Figure 2: Heart failure pathophysiology. From Packer M: The neurohormonal hypothesis: a theory to explain the mechanism of disease progression in heart failure. *J Am Coll Cardiol* 1992;20:248-254.

the volume loads on the heart. If sustained over time, this load increase will stimulate remodeling. However, many of the agents are also able to promote remodeling by their direct stimulation of either growth or activation of heart cells. In cardiomyocytes, neurohormonal agents promote cell hypertrophy and expression of the fetal gene pattern, with a resultant alteration in several important myocyte proteins. In fibroblasts, neurohormonal activation increases cell replication, migration, and production of ECM proteins, such as fibronectin and collagen. Thus, neurohormonal agents have direct (growth-related) as well as indirect (increased load) effects that promote the remodeling process.

There is also evidence that a great deal of crosstalk occurs between the neurohormonal systems, so activation of one system often results in enhanced activation of other systems. For example, one effect of NE is stimulating the release of renin activity from the juxtaglomerular apparatus of the kidney. However, not all of the neurohormonal agents that are increased in the failing heart promote cardiac remodeling. Elevated wall stress within the heart increases production and release of factors such as atrial natriuretic peptide (ANP) and brain natriuretic peptide (BNP), which have both vasodilatory and diuretic properties. The natriuretic peptides appear to inhibit release of growth-promoting neurohormones, such as ET, and they act directly to inhibit growth and activation of cardiac cells. Thus, they tend to regulate the adverse consequences of other agents that are activated both locally and systemically, such as the renin-angiotensin and sympathetic nervous systems. Unfortunately, there is an imbalance between the factors that promote remodeling and those that inhibit it, so although the natriuretic peptides may modulate the process somewhat, the net effect of neurohormonal activation is to stimulate cardiac growth.

Systemic neurohormonal activation is a consequence of hemodynamic perturbations that cause a reduction in perfusion pressure, while local activation of systems within the heart can be initiated either by altered hemodynamics (usually associated with increased ventricular filling pressures) or in response to myocardial damage. Systemic neurohormonal activation begins early after damage to the heart occurs. After an MI, there is evidence of widespread neurohormonal activation that probably develops as a way to maintain perfusion pressure for vital organs. With resolution of the acute event, some of these systemic factors become quiescent. However, activation of systems (eg, the intracardiac renin-angiotensin system) also occurs within the heart.

Persistent activation of neurohormonal systems, both systemically and locally within the heart, results in increased load and sustained stimulation of cardiac cells, both of which drive the remodeling process. Results from a survey of neurohormones sampled from the blood of patients with LV dysfunction in the SOLVD program are helpful in explaining both the pattern and importance of neurohormonal activation in the development of heart failure. Patients enrolled in SOLVD had evidence of LV dysfunction, manifested by an EF <0.35. Subjects without evidence of symptomatic heart failure were enrolled in the prevention arm of the study, while patients with the usual signs and symptoms of heart failure were enrolled in the treatment arm. As depicted in Figure 3, evidence showed an increase in the levels of the neurohormones sampled in the asymptomatic prevention arm patients. In the symptomatic treatment arm patients, further activation of these systems became evident. The results of this study provide evidence that neurohormonal activation precedes the development of overt heart failure. Since these factors tend to promote growth, these findings suggest that early neurohormonal activation plays a causative role in the remodeling process. The results also show that as heart failure progresses, further neurohormonal activation occurs, indicating an intensification of the process.

Perhaps the most persuasive evidence that neurohormonal activation causes remodeling comes from a substantial body of evidence from large-scale clinical trials in which neurohormonal blocking agents, such as angiotensin-converting enzyme (ACE) inhibitors and β-blockers, were given to patients with heart failure. These studies are reviewed extensively in the respective chapters dealing with these agents. However, the results demonstrate that neurohormonal blocking agents are associated with inhibition of the remodeling process. This effect appears to be related to the favorable impact that these agents have on the clinical course of heart failure patients and pro-

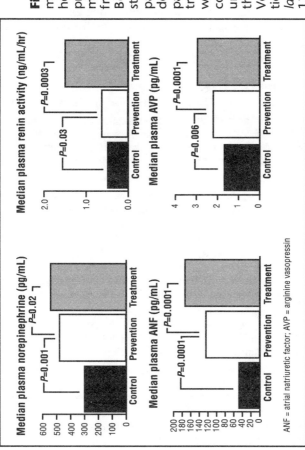

Figure 3: Neurohormonal activation in heart failure (SOLVD prevention and treatment trials). Adapted from Francis GS, Benedict C, Johnstone DE, et al: Comparison of neuroendocrine activation in patients with left ventricular dysfunction with and without congestive heart failure: a sub-study of the Studies of Left Ventricular Dysfunction (SOLVD). *Circulation* 1990; 82:1724-1729.

ANF = atrial natriuretic factor; AVP = arginine vasopressin

vides the basis for the use of drugs, such as ACE inhibitors and β-blockers, for the treatment of heart failure.

The knowledge that remodeling plays such a critical role in the progression of heart failure has important implications for the development of future therapies. A variety of new approaches (both drugs and mechanical devices) are being evaluated as prospective treatments for heart failure. The close association between the effects of a therapy in preventing or reversing cardiac remodeling and reduced risk of future events suggests the possibility that the effects of an intervention on the remodeling process could be considered a surrogate end point for clinical efficacy.

Suggested Readings

Beltrami CA, Finato N, Rocco M, et al: Structural basis of end-stage failure in ischemic cardiomyopathy in humans. *Circulation* 1994; 89:151-163.

Braunwald E, Bristow MR: Congestive heart failure: fifty years of progress. *Circulation* 2000;102(suppl 4):IV14-IV23.

Chien KR: Stress pathways and heart failure. *Cell* 1999;98:555-558.

Cohn JN, Ferrari R, Sharpe N: Cardiac remodeling—concepts and clinical implications: a consensus paper from an international forum on cardiac remodeling. On behalf of the International Forum on Cardiac Remodeling. *J Am Coll Cardiol* 2000;35:569-582.

Francis GS, Benedict C, Johnstone DE, et al: Comparison of neuroendocrine activation in patients with left ventricular dysfunction with and without congestive heart failure. A substudy of the Studies of Left Ventricular Dysfunction (SOLVD). *Circulation* 1990; 82:1724-1729.

Francis GS, McDonald KM, Cohn JN: Neurohormonal activation in preclinical heart failure. Remodeling and the potential for intervention. *Circulation* 1993;87(suppl 4):IV90-IV96.

Greenberg B, Quinones MA, Koilpillai C, et al: Effects of long-term enalapril therapy on cardiac structure and function in patients with left ventricular dysfunction. Results of the SOLVD echocardiography substudy. *Circulation* 1995;91:2573-2581.

Hunter JJ, Chien KR: Signaling pathways for cardiac hypertrophy and failure. *N Engl J Med* 1999;341:1276-1283.

Katz AM: The cardiomyopathy of overload: an unnatural growth response in the hypertrophied heart. *Ann Intern Med* 1994;121: 363-371.

Levy D, Anderson KM, Savage DD, et al: Risk of ventricular arrhythmias in left ventricular hypertrophy: the Framingham heart study. *Am J Cardiol* 1987;60:560-565.

Levy D, Garrison RJ, Savage DD, et al: Prognostic implications of echocardiographically determined left ventricular mass in the Framingham heart study. *N Engl J Med* 1990;322:1561-1566.

Lorell BH, Carabello BA: Left ventricular hypertrophy: pathogenesis, detection, and prognosis. *Circulation* 2000;102:470-479.

McKay RG, Pfeffer MA, Pasternak RC, et al: Left ventricular remodeling after myocardial infarction: a corollary to infarct expansion. *Circulation* 1986;74:693-702.

Mercadier JJ: Progression from cardiac hypertrophy to heart failure. In: Hosenpud JD, Greenberg BH, eds. *Congestive Heart Failure. Pathophysiology, Diagnosis and Comprehensive Approach to Management*, 2nd ed. Philadelphia, Lippincott Williams and Wilkins, 2000, pp 41-65.

Packer M: The neurohormonal hypothesis: a theory to explain the mechanism of disease progression in heart failure. *J Am Coll Cardiol* 1992;20:248-254.

Poole-Wilson PA: Heart failure. *Med Intern* 1985;2:866-871.

Quinones MA, Greenberg BH, Kopelen HA, et al: Echocardiographic predictors of clinical outcome in patients with left ventricular dysfunction enrolled in the SOLVD registry and trials: significance of left ventricular hypertrophy. Studies of Left Ventricular Dysfunction. *J Am Coll Cardiol* 2000;35:1237-1244.

Rouleau JL, De Champlain J, Klein M, et al: Activation of neurohumoral systems in postinfarction left ventricular dysfunction. *J Am Coll Cardiol* 1993;22:390-398.

Sabbah HN: Apoptotic cell death in heart failure. *Cardiovasc Res* 2000;45:704-712.

Sabbah HN, Sharov VG, Goldstein S: Cell death, tissue hypoxia and the progression of heart failure. *Heart Fail Rev* 2000;5: 131-138.

Sadoshima J, Izumo S: Molecular characterization of angiotensin II-induced hypertrophy of cardiac myocytes and hyperplasia of cardiac fibroblasts. Critical role of the AT_1 receptor subtype. *Circ Res* 1993;73:413-423.

Schrier RW, Abraham WT: Hormones and hemodynamics in heart failure. *N Engl J Med* 1999;341:577-585.

Schwartz K, Carrier L, Mercadier JJ, et al: Molecular phenotype of the hypertrophied and failing myocardium. *Circulation* 1993;87(suppl 7):VII5-VII10.

St. John Sutton M, Pfeffer MA, Plappert T, et al: Quantitative two-dimensional echocardiographic measurements are major predicators of adverse cardiovascular events after acute myocardial infarction. The protective effects of captopril. *Circulation* 1994; 89:68-75.

Sullivan JM, Vander Zwaag RV, el-Zeky F, et al: Left ventricular hypertrophy: effect on survival. *J Am Coll Cardiol* 1993;22: 508-513.

Sutton MG, Sharpe N: Left ventricular remodeling after myocardial infarction: pathophysiology and therapy. *Circulation* 2000;101:2981-2988.

Vasan RS, Larson MG, Benjamin EJ, et al: Left ventricular dilatation and the risk of congestive heart failure in people without myocardial infarction. *N Engl J Med* 1997;336:1350-1355.

Weber KT: Extracellular matrix remodeling in heart failure: a role for de novo angiotensin II generation. *Circulation* 1997;96: 4065-4082.

White HD, Norris RM, Brown MA, et al: Left ventricular end-systolic volume as the major determinant of survival after recovery from myocardial infarction. *Circulation* 1987;76:44-51.

 Chapter **2**

Diagnosis and Evaluation of Chronic Heart Failure

Heart failure, a complex clinical syndrome diagnosed by the presence of a symptom complex derived from impaired cardiac function, may be either acute or chronic. The 'classic' presentation of acute, severe heart failure evokes an image of a patient with pink frothy pulmonary edema fluid, diffuse pulmonary rales, and overt cardiogenic shock. However, identical hemodynamic measurements without extreme symptoms or physical examination signs are commonly found in the patient with chronic heart failure, reflecting a slow and insidious onset. Consequently, while the acute presentation is easily recognized, classic symptoms of chronic heart failure (dyspnea, fatigue) are frequently misinterpreted in clinical practice. This chapter focuses on the diagnosis and evaluation of the patient with chronic heart failure.

Heart failure is a preventable disease. Early identification and treatment of left ventricular (LV) dysfunction saves lives. Therefore, patients at risk for the development of heart failure should be assessed periodically for attributable symptoms. Common independent risk factors for chronic heart failure include aging, atherosclerotic

Table 1: Heart Failure Risk Factors

- Aging
- Coronary artery disease
- Hypertension
- Left ventricular hypertrophy
- Diabetes mellitus
- Obesity

coronary disease, diabetes, hypertension, LV hypertrophy, and obesity (Table 1). Clinicians should note that impaired LV function may, in fact, be asymptomatic, although slowly progressive symptoms may be rationalized as a 'normal' consequence of aging or attributed to poor physical conditioning.

The American College of Cardiology and American Heart Association Task Force of Practice Guidelines have created a novel 4-stage grading system for chronic heart failure (Table 2). These guidelines have been officially endorsed by the Heart Failure Society of America and the International Society of Heart and Lung Transplantation. The staging system focuses on heart failure as a progressive disorder rather than a symptomatic disease. The evolution and progression of heart failure are characterized by four stages of disease progression, starting with asymptomatic patients at risk. In these patients, left ventricular dysfunction arises from myocardial injury or stress. Once sufficient injury has occurred, the process of heart failure generally continues, even in the absence of further insult to the heart. The mechanism of this progression, known as *cardiac remodeling*, manifests as a change in the geometry of the left ventricle, including chamber dilation, increasing sphericity, and hypertrophy. These morphologic changes increase hemodynamic stress on the walls of the failing heart, further depress mechanical performance, and promote continued remodeling. Not all patients progress sequentially through these stages, although most do. This staging system allows the use of specific treatments targeted at each stage for the purpose of reducing morbidity and mortality.

Symptoms

Heart failure is the symptomatic manifestation of the heart's inability to generate sufficient cardiac output to meet the metabolic needs of body tissues without or despite intracardiac hemodynamic perturbation. Symptoms commonly observed in chronic heart failure patients are typically categorized as *congestive* or *low cardiac output* (Table 3), but they may coexist regardless of category. The adjective *congestive* is most appropriate when symptoms or signs of systemic or pulmonary fluid volume overload exist.

Although it is a common misperception, the diagnosis of chronic heart failure does not indicate the underlying etiology or nature of cardiac dysfunction (systolic vs diastolic). Symptoms consistent with chronic heart failure are often observed in noncardiac conditions, such as primary pulmonary hypertension and cor pulmonale. The differential diagnosis of heart failure is shown in Table 4.

Despite well-known subjective limitations, symptoms are traditionally classified according to the New York Heart Association (NYHA) Classification (Table 5). NYHA Class I patients have no perceived limitation of physical activity. In NYHA Class II patients, physical exertion produces heart failure symptoms (eg, fatigue, dyspnea). NYHA Class III patients are comfortable at rest but develop heart failure symptoms with low levels of activity, such as those required for the activities of daily living. NYHA Class IV patients experience resting symptoms. Classes II and III are often difficult to distinguish and have been further subcategorized into NYHA II A/B and III A/B, reflecting early vs late symptom manifestations in each stage.

Table 2: American College of Cardiology/American Heart Association Stages of Heart Failure

Stage	Description
A	Patients at high risk of developing heart failure because of the presence of conditions that are strongly associated with the development of heart failure. Such patients have no identified structural or functional abnormalities of the pericardium, myocardium, or cardiac valves and have never shown signs or symptoms of heart failure.
B	Patients who have developed structural heart disease that is strongly associated with the development of heart failure but who have never shown signs or symptoms of heart failure.
C	Patients who have current or prior symptoms of heart failure associated with underlying structural heart disease.
D	Patients with advanced structural heart disease and marked symptoms of heart failure at rest despite maximal medical therapy and who require specialized interventions.

Examples

Systemic hypertension; coronary artery disease; diabetes mellitus; history of cardiotoxic drug therapy or alcohol abuse; personal history of rheumatic fever; family history of cardiomyopathy

Left ventricular hypertrophy or fibrosis; left ventricular dilatation or hypocontractility; asymptomatic valvular heart disease; previous myocardial infarction

Dyspnea or fatigue due to left ventricular systolic dysfunction; ventricular systolic dysfunction; asymptomatic patients who are undergoing treatment for prior symptoms of heart failure

Patients who are frequently hospitalized for heart failure and cannot be safely discharged from the hospital; patients in the hospital awaiting heart transplantation; patients at home receiving continuous intravenous support for symptom relief or being supported with a mechanical circulatory assist device; patients in a hospice setting for the management of heart failure

Table 3: Common Symptoms of Chronic Heart Failure

Congestive

- Dyspnea (rest or exertional)
- Paroxysmal nocturnal dyspnea
- Abdominal or epigastric discomfort
- Nausea or anorexia
- Pedal/leg edema
- Sleep disturbance (anxiety or air hunger)
- Orthopnea
- Cough (recumbent or exertional)
- Abdominal bloating (ascites)
- Early satiety
- Weight gain (rapid)
- Chest tightness or discomfort

Low Cardiac Output

- Easy fatigability
- Nausea or anorexia
- Poor energy level or endurance
- Weight loss, unexplained
- Impaired concentration or memory
- Sleep disturbance (Cheyne-Stokes respiration)
- Malaise
- Early satiety
- Decreased exercise tolerance
- Muscle wasting or weakness
- Daytime oliguria with recumbent nocturia

Table 4: Differential Diagnosis of Chronic Heart Failure

Dyspnea +/- Edema

- Pulmonary parenchymal disease, chronic obstructive or interstitial
- Pulmonary thromboembolic disease
- Cor pulmonale
- Pulmonary venous occlusive disease
- Primary pulmonary hypertension
- Other secondary pulmonary hypertension
- Exertional asthma
- Severe anemia
- Mitral stenosis
- Neuromuscular disease
- Constrictive pericarditis
- Metabolic causes (acidosis)

Edema +/- Dyspnea

- Nephrotic syndrome
- Cirrhosis
- Venous insufficiency
- Combined vascular insufficiency
- Lymphedema
- Adverse medication effect

In assessing NYHA symptom class, clinicians should try to maintain a frame of reference to the typical activities of an age- and gender-matched normal individual. In each patient, symptom classification is subject to fluctuation. The NYHA classification describing the patient's baseline *compensated* state is most useful for the purpose of titration of medical

Table 5: New York Heart Association Function Classification of Chronic Heart Failure

Class	Symptoms
I	No perceived limitation of physical activity
II A/B	Symptoms with moderate physical exertion
III A/B	Symptoms with low levels of physical exertion (ie, those for activities of daily living)
IV	Resting symptoms

A = early stage; B = late stage

therapy and for determining prognosis. Despite its limitations, NYHA symptom classification is still useful as a surrogate predictor of clinical outcome. Generally, patients with NYHA Class IV symptoms have significantly worsened survival (40% to 60% annual mortality risk) compared with NYHA Class I/IIA patients (5% to 10% annual mortality risk). Interestingly, there is no correlation between symptom class and LV ejection fraction (LVEF).

Medical History and Physical Examination

In a patient with symptoms of chronic heart failure, the medical history and physical examination should focus on determining the etiology of cardiac dysfunction and other factors contributing to symptom precipitation. In many cases, treatment of the initiating disease process may improve cardiac function.

Coronary Artery Disease (CAD)

In the United States, 60% to 75% of patients in clinical trials of heart failure and systolic LV dysfunction have underlying ischemic cardiomyopathy. Patients with both heart failure and risk factors for CAD should be evaluated for the presence of CAD, as revascularization may be appropriate.

Hypertension

Hypertension is a risk factor for the development of CAD, but it is also an independent risk factor for the development of heart failure. In patient populations with heart failure and preserved systolic LV function, a history of hypertension is extremely common. Patients on chronic antihypertensive therapy with long-standing inadequate resting or exertional blood pressure control, those with recorded systolic blood pressures >200 mm Hg, and those who have been treated for hypertensive urgencies or crises are likely to have hypertensive cardiomyopathy (increased LV mass and wall thickness, reflecting myocardial hypertrophy). In late stages, hypertensive heart failure can result in progressive LV chamber dilation, wall thinning, and impairment of systolic function.

Endocrinopathy

Diabetes. Cardiomyopathy in association with long-standing diabetes has been described (excluding CAD), although typically in association with additional end-organ damage. Diabetic amyloid deposition in the myocardium may partly initially contribute to diastolic myocardial relaxation abnormalities, followed by systolic ventricular impairment. Additionally, uncontrolled diabetes promotes decompensation of chronic heart failure related to hyperosmolar stress and increased infection risk.

Thyroid disease. Asymptomatic or symptomatic thyroid conditions related to either hypo- or hyperthyroidism can induce or exacerbate underlying myocardial dysfunction, mediated by isoform alterations in myocardial myosin.

Growth hormone excess, pheochromocytoma, hyperaldosteronism, Cushing's syndrome. These conditions are fairly rare, but treatable.

Recent Pregnancy

Heart failure occurring within months after the delivery of a child in a woman with no prior history of heart disease, preeclampsia, or other identified etiology of cardiomyopathy is likely to be caused by peripartum cardiomyopathy. In this setting, the natural history is similar to that of idiopathic cardiomyopathy.

Family History

Researchers estimate that nearly 10% to 15% of heart failure patients may have a family history of cardiomyopathy. A family history of sudden unexplained (cardiac) death should, therefore, be sought in all patients. The most detailed genetic linkages reflect variants of hypertrophic cardiomyopathy. Additional inheritable cardiomyopathies, such as hemochromocytosis or muscular dystrophies, should be considered in the appropriate setting.

Substance Abuse

A careful history of the quantity of alcohol consumed and the frequency of consumption should be obtained from each patient. Generally, chronic consumption of ethanol for a prolonged duration (typically several years) and the exclusion of other causes are required to attribute a heart failure diagnosis to alcoholic cardiomyopathy. Cardiomyopathy has also been observed in association with chronic amphetamine and/or cocaine use. These agents may cause direct myocardial toxicity or affect ventricular function through either small- or large-vessel CAD or vascular dysfunction. Current and former intravenous drug users may present with progressive valvular heart disease from prior infectious endocarditis. Patients with a lifestyle risk of intravenous substance abuse are also at risk for hepatitis C viral infection, which has been associated with a dilated cardiomyopathy.

Drugs and Toxins

Chemotherapeutic agents. Doxorubicin (Adriamycin®) and other anthracyclines, cyclophosphamide (Cytoxan®, Neosar®), and several other chemotherapeutic agents may cause acute (peak bolus dose) toxic myocardial damage. Cumulative dose toxicity represents a more chronic form of injury and is infrequent with anthracyclines at doses less than 400 to 450 mg/m^2. However, subclinical myocardial injury that occurs during drug administration may result in progressive ventricular remodeling and late-onset heart failure months to years later. Certain risk factors (advanced age, concomitant mediastinal irradiation, preexisting myocardial disease) increase the likelihood of myocardial toxicity. Chemotherapy-related cardiomyopathy, however, represents a diagnosis of exclusion when heart failure is of late onset. In addition to direct myocardial cellular injury, an eosinophilic myocarditis has been reported in association with interleukin-2 (IL-2) administration.

Inflammatory myocardial disease. Several common pharmacologic agents have potential cardiotoxic effects (eg, high-dose catecholamine administration). Other drugs have been associated with either a direct toxic or hypersensitivity (allergic) eosinophilic myocarditis. Sulfa- or sulfur-containing drugs predominate, although others include such commonly used agents as quinidine (Quinidex®, Quinaglute®), hydralazine (Apresoline®), amitriptyline (eg, Elavil®), spironolactone (Aldactone®), acetazolamide (eg, Diamox™), isoniazid (eg, Laniazid®), penicillin, amphotericin B (Fungizone®), phenothiazines, carbamazepine (eg, Tegretol®), and phenytoin (eg, Dilantin®).

Negatively inotropic medications. Agents such as calcium-channel blockers, (full-dose) β-blockers, and most antiarrhythmic drugs that depress cardiac function may precipitate heart failure symptoms. However, this probably represents an exacerbation of preexisting or subclinical cardiac dysfunction of another etiology.

Medications causing fluid retention. Institution of agents that promote avid sodium and water retention may also precipitate congestive heart failure symptoms in patients with preexisting or subclinical cardiac dysfunction. These drugs include, but are not limited to, nonsteroidal anti-inflammatory drugs (NSAIDs), corticosteroids, COX-2 inhibitors, peripherally acting α-blockers for the treatment of benign prostatic hypertrophy, hormone replacement or modulation therapy, and several of the newer glitazone class of insulin-sensitizing drugs. Over-the-counter or naturoceutical products may also contribute to water retention.

Other toxins. Lead, arsenic, and cobalt are toxic metals that can cause progressive and dose-related myocardial dysfunction when consumed. Endogenous toxins that depress myocardial function are classically seen in uremia and sepsis (tumor necrosis factor-α).

Connective Tissue and Other Systemic Disorders

Patients with systemic lupus erythematosus, scleroderma, polymyositis, and other connective tissue disorders may develop an associated cardiomyopathy with heart failure. In these conditions, as well as in granulomatous disorders (ie, sarcoidosis) and infiltrative disease (amyloidosis), the typical patient presents with heart failure and initially preserved systolic ventricular function.

Myocarditis

Some forms of myocarditis are catastrophic in their initial presentation, such as fulminant viral myocarditis and giant cell myocarditis. More commonly, postviral myocarditis is characterized by a subacute onset, reflecting a gradual deterioration after resolution of the acute viral syndrome. At least 20 viruses have been causally associated with clinical evidence of myocarditis, generally those causing upper respiratory or gastrointestinal syndromes. Heart failure caused by HIV-related cardiomyopathy is an uncommon presentation of HIV infection but is easily screened for in appropriate patients. Other infectious etiologies of myocarditis (eg, parasitic, chagasic, viral, rickettsial, bacterial, and fungal) are extremely uncommon.

Metabolic deficiencies

Beriberi (thiamine deficiency) may appear in individuals on fad diets or on long-term, high-dose diuretics and in hospitalized patients receiving only salt or glucose replacement without proper nutritional support. Inherited or acquired metabolic deficiencies (carnitine, coenzyme Q-10) are rare.

Hemoglobinopathies

Patients with certain hemoglobinopathies, such as thalassemia and sickle cell disease, who have undergone repeated transfusions can develop heart failure related to myocardial iron overload accompanying a high-output state derived from chronic anemia.

High-Output States

Hyperthyroidism, severe chronic anemia, large intrinsic or iatrogenic arteriovenous shunts, Paget's disease, and sepsis may result in high-output failure.

Valvular Heart Disease

Although this category represented the most common etiology of heart failure in the early Framingham studies, valvular disease is now more often a consequence of ventricular dilation than a cause. However, a history of rheumatic or other valvular disease can be important in defining the etiology of the patient's cardiac dysfunction, as the physical findings may be muted by low cardiac output or high filling pressures.

Idiopathic Etiology

When ventricular dysfunction presents without identifiable etiology or specific causative factor, the term *idiopathic cardiomyopathy* is generally used. This etiology represents approximately 10% to 20% of patient populations with heart failure.

Physical Examination: Hemodynamic and Volume Assessment

Physical signs of chronic heart failure are often subtle and, like radiographic findings, have poor positive and negative predictive value in estimating intracardiac hemodynamics. For example, patients may have a marked elevation of pulmonary capillary wedge pressure (left atrial pressure) without manifesting pulmonary rales, if the he-

Table 6: Physical Examination Findings and Typically Associated Hemodynamic Perturbations in Chronic Heart Failure

Reduced Cardiac Output

- Resting tachycardia
- Pulsus alternans
- Cachexia
- Cheyne-Stokes respiration (with or without apnea)
- Low carotid pulse volume
- Cool or vasoconstricted extremities
- Altered mentation (somnolence, confusion)

Volume and/or Diastolic Pressure Overload

- Jugular venous distention
- Abdominojugular reflux
- Ascites
- S3
- Hepatomegaly
- Pleural effusion
- Dependent edema
- Loud pulmonic closure sound
- Pulmonary rales

Nonspecific Hemodynamic Correlation

- Cardiomegaly
- S4
- Accessory respiratory muscle use
- Wheezing
- Subxiphoid impulse
- Abnormal apical impulse
- Tachypnea
- Parasternal lift

modynamic perturbation was slowly achieved. However, while physical signs in chronic heart failure have diagnostic limitations, certain abnormalities have profound prognostic implications. For example, the presence of elevated jugular venous pressure, rales, and an S3 in a patient with chronic heart failure imply a much more adverse prognosis.

Common physical findings in chronic heart failure with correlative hemodynamic derangements are listed in Table 6. Resting tachycardia is a frequent manifestation of the hyperadrenergic state, designed as an intrinsic compensatory mechanism to preserve resting cardiac output. A resting heart rate >120 to 130 beats/min may suggest tachycardia-induced cardiomyopathy. However, in most patients with heart failure, resting tachycardia represents a compensatory response to maintain cardiac output and tissue perfusion in the setting of clinical decompensation.

Venous Inspection

Marked jugular venous distention (>15 cm of water) or a lesser degree of elevation with Kussmaul's physiology (absence of an inspiratory pressure drop) indicates restrictive right heart filling. This may reveal the etiology of cardiac dysfunction (restrictive/constrictive disease) or merely reflect severe biventricular failure with volume overload. Massive jugular v-waves suggest severe tricuspid regurgitation and, therefore, either primary or secondary pulmonary hypertension. Abdominojugular reflux is frequently demonstrated in volume overload states. Hepatic enlargement or tenderness secondary to right heart congestion should be sought; hepatic pulsatility suggests significant tricuspid regurgitation.

Arterial Inspection

Carotid upstrokes should be assessed for delay, indicating hemodynamically significant aortic stenosis. Bifid and dynamic carotid pulsation may indicate hypertrophic cardiomyopathy. Carotid bruits or signs of peripheral arterial disease increase the likelihood of associated atherosclerotic CAD. Low-volume impulses are often palpated in a low cardiac output state. Pulsus alternans implies low cardiac output and severe systolic ventricular dysfunction.

43

Peripheral Perfusion

Assessment or palpation of warm extremities with good capillary refill generally reflects an adequate resting cardiac output. Cool, vasoconstricted extremities with or without mild cyanosis imply significantly reduced cardiac output, with increased systemic vascular resistance as a compensatory mechanism to preserve vital organ perfusion.

Marked lower-extremity edema without an elevation in jugular venous pressure should prompt an evaluation for chronic venous insufficiency or thrombosis, hypoalbuminemia, or hepatic disease. In the setting of jugular distention, ascites disproportionate to lower-extremity edema may suggest restrictive/constrictive cardiomyopathy or severe tricuspid regurgitation.

Chest Palpation/Percussion

Chest palpation/percussion reveals the presence of cardiac enlargement by localizing the apical impulse. A forceful point of maximal impulse (PMI) with an S4 gallop suggests LV hypertrophy, while a parasternal heave typically suggests right ventricular hypertrophy and enlargement. A loud or palpable pulmonic closure sound may be heard in patients with pulmonary hypertension. An inferolaterally displaced PMI represents significant ventricular dilation and in the presence of a dyskinetic apical impulse is a sensitive, but not specific, finding of underlying ischemic cardiomyopathy. A displaced PMI accompanied by an S3 gallop is the most specific finding for systolic LV dysfunction.

Auscultation

Cardiac murmurs, including aortic stenosis, aortic regurgitation, mitral stenosis, and mitral regurgitation, may indicate a surgically remedial etiology of heart failure. However, an elevation in ventricular end-diastolic pressure or a reduced cardiac output may soften regurgitant and stenotic murmurs. Auscultation of the lung fields seeks evidence of pleural effusion, rales, or wheezes (cardiac asthma). A more sensitive but subtle finding in chronic heart failure is limited inspiratory diaphragmatic descent, reflecting decreased lung compliance caused by an increase in interstitial lung water. Gallops can be variable and may derive from either the right or left ventricle. However, a left-sided S3 is classically associated with systolic ventricular dysfunction and impairment of early ventricular filling, which is more likely in LV volume overload. An S4 is more likely related to an increase in end-diastolic pressure/loading conditions with ventricular relaxation abnormality.

Diagnostic Evaluation

The clinical diagnosis of heart failure and its suspected pathophysiology must be confirmed by objective evaluation. All patients with symptoms or signs consistent with heart failure should undergo a formal assessment of cardiac function. Specifically, the LVEF and wall motion should be evaluated by echocardiography with Doppler imaging or radionuclide ventriculography. These testing modalities can also evaluate ventricular diastolic filling pattern and rate and, therefore, can indicate predominant systolic or diastolic dysfunction, or both. A diagnostic treatment algorithm emphasizing the importance of evaluation and treatment for underlying CAD is shown in Figure 1.

Echocardiography is fast and accurate and yields additional information, including cardiac chamber dimensions, ejection fraction, wall thickness, myocardial tissue characterization, and valvular structure and function. Doppler interrogation adds an accurate estimation of valvular disease severity. Doppler peak velocity evaluation allows estimation of hemodynamics when the jugular venous pressure and arterial blood pressure are known. Further, derivation of systolic flow rates enables an assessment of LV dP/dT and cardiac output, while diastolic function is delineated through analysis of transmitral and pulmonary venous flow.

After confirming the diagnosis and character of ventricular dysfunction, the next step is to determine the etiology of chronic heart failure. When CAD is suspected,

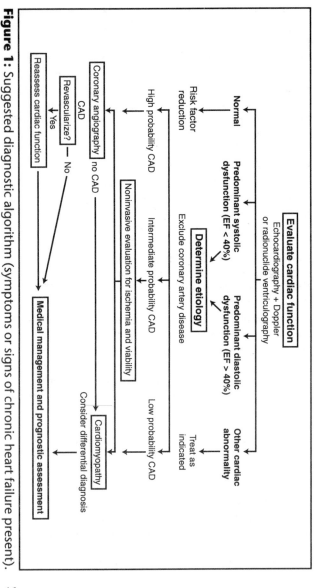

Figure 1: Suggested diagnostic algorithm (symptoms or signs of chronic heart failure present).

46

noninvasive stress testing for perfusion abnormalities or direct coronary angiography should be performed. In the absence of active or reversible ischemia, an assessment of myocardial viability should be considered, as reversible or treatable factors for ongoing myocardial injury must not be overlooked.

The electrocardiogram (EKG) is not a useful screening tool for assessing either the presence of heart failure or its etiology, but it should be obtained. Left atrial enlargement, atrial fibrillation, LV hypertrophy, old myocardial infarction, left bundle branch block, left axis deviation, and repolarization abnormalities are extremely common findings on EKG. A low QRS voltage or a pseudoinfarction pattern may direct attention to otherwise occult primary or secondary myocardial disease, such as amyloidosis.

Baseline two-view chest radiography should also be performed, as it provides information on general cardiac chamber size, great vessel enlargement or tortuosity, abnormal thoracic calcification, and concomitant lung parenchymal or vascular disease, including pulmonary venous congestion and pruning. The posteroanterior chest radiograph alone will not demonstrate cardiomegaly in the setting of isolated LV enlargement.

Additional testing commonly performed on patients with the clinical syndrome of heart failure includes a baseline screening laboratory assessment consisting of a standard chemistry profile with renal and hepatic function, a sensitive thyroid-stimulating hormone (TSH) assay, a complete blood count (CBC), and other blood tests, as indicated by the history and physical examination. Patients without fasting lipid profiles should have them performed. In diabetic patients, measurement of glycosylated hemoglobin provides a sense of recent glycemic control, a risk factor in worsening heart failure symptoms.

Because significant ventricular dysfunction may produce few symptoms, and because symptoms consistent with heart failure have a substantial diagnostic differential, a simple yet inexpensive and accurate screening test that confirms or excludes a diagnosis of heart failure is appealing. Derived from ventricular myocardium, brain natriuretic peptide (BNP, or n-terminal pro-BNP) assays hold promise for this purpose. An abnormal (elevated) BNP level seems to be predictive of any perturbation in ventricular filling pressure or increased wall stress. The role of BNP in the clinical evaluation and management of chronic heart failure patients remains to be more completely defined. BNP testing may be best used in cases where the diagnosis remains uncertain after the history, physical examination, and available conventional noninvasive diagnostic tests have been performed. For example, the assay may be particularly helpful in the rapid evaluation of acute dyspnea in the emergency department or urgent-care outpatient setting. The role of BNP in helping monitor the response to therapy and in screening high-risk populations is being evaluated.

Additional Useful Tests

Standard exercise stress testing (bicycle or treadmill) provides an objective assessment of a patient's functional exercise limitation and hemodynamic response to exercise. It also helps screen for evidence of exercise-induced arrhythmia or ischemia (angina); however, the EKG is typically nondiagnostic for ischemia in patients with heart failure due to resting abnormalities or medication effects.

However, when combined with either echocardiography or radionuclide ventriculography and perfusion imaging, exercise or pharmacologic stress testing more accurately establishes the presence of coronary disease by identifying regions of scarring, inducible ischemia, and/or myocardial viability. Maximal exercise testing with concomitant measurement of oxygen consumption is exceedingly useful in estimating heart failure prognosis. The latter also serves as a guide for an individualized exercise rehabilitation prescription.

Right heart catheterization is most appropriate for patients whose filling pressures and/or cardiac output remain uncertain after physical examination and noninvasive assessment. Additionally, invasive hemodynamic assessment should be considered in patients intolerant of standard therapy or in patients for whom medical therapy has failed to achieve symptomatic relief. Such patients are frequently candidates for inotrope or inodilator therapy.

Noninvasive evaluation of hemodynamic parameters by bioimpedance plethysmography or oscillometric wave analysis may be a surrogate for pulmonary arterial catheterization. However, the accuracy, reproducibility, and clinical utility of these diagnostic modalities in heart failure are incompletely defined.

In the absence of sustained or symptomatic ventricular tachycardia, unexplained syncope, or survived sudden death, routine electrophysiologic testing has little diagnostic value, particularly in patients with ischemic cardiomyopathy. Endomyocardial biopsy is rarely necessary to establish the etiology of chronic heart failure, but it provides definitive pathologic evidence for several disorders, including primary cardiac amyloidosis, giant cell myocarditis, active cardiac sarcoidosis, and eosinophilic myocarditis.

Prognostic Assessment

The evaluation of a patient with chronic heart failure is incomplete without an initial and periodic assessment of prognosis that encompasses patient demographics, symptoms, and objective clinical parameters. A summary of prognostic indicators can be found in Table 7. After institution and titration of standard medical therapy, residual symptoms or persistent adverse prognostic indicators should prompt an assessment for additional therapeutic options and interventions.

Symptoms correlate well with prognosis in systolic LV dysfunction. Despite standard medical therapy, patients with persistent NYHA Class IV symptoms have an an-

Table 7: Prognostic Indicators in Systolic Ventricular Dysfunction*

Patient demographics	Age (older)
	Gender (?male>female)
	Race (?African American>white)
Comorbidities	Diabetes
	Pulmonary hypertension
	Systemic hypertension
	Significant renal or hepatic dysfunction
	Morbid obesity
	Cachexia
	Thyroid disease
Symptoms	NYHA classification (IV>III>II>I)
Ejection fraction	Left ventricular ejection fraction (lower)
	Right ventricular ejection fraction (biventricular>left only)
Left ventricular morphology	Size and volume (larger)
	Shape (globular)
	Mass (increased)
Exercise capacity	VO_2 max (lower)
	Exertional hypotension
	6-minute walk distance (<305 m)

nual mortality rate of 40% to 60%, compared with 5% to 10% in NYHA Class I/II patients. However, NYHA class and objective parameters are not necessarily congruent, which is illustrated by the well-documented lack of correlation between symptoms and LVEF or LVEF and exercise performance in patients with systolic ventricular

Serum sodium	Hyponatremia (<135 mg/dL)
Arrhythmias	Atrial or ventricular (any)
Doppler echo	Restrictive pattern in mitral inflow or pulmonary venous waveform
Neurohormone/ cytokine elevation	Norepinephrine Renin Angiotensin II Aldosterone Natriuretic factors/peptides Endothelin Tumor necrosis factor-α

* The variables listed to the right of the bolded categories provide prognostic information in chronic heart failure. The presence of a question mark (?) indicates a variable that has been suggested but not prospectively demonstrated as a prognostic indicator. The parenthetical information describes the parameter or directional trend reflecting a more adverse prognosis.

dysfunction. Each variable examined has independent predictive power.

An LVEF of 30% to 35% reflects a high risk group, particularly among patients with ischemic cardiomyopathy. The greater the degree of decreased contractility (lower ejection fraction), the greater the mortality risk.

Table 8: Key Features of Heart Failure Diagnosis and Evaluation

For all patients at risk

- Recognize and modify risk factors for chronic heart failure

- Identify heart failure symptoms when present

- Evaluate for signs of heart failure on physical examination

For patients with symptoms or signs

- Determine nature and extent of left ventricular dysfunction

- Identify etiology and exacerbating comorbidities

- Evaluate prognosis

Right ventricular systolic dysfunction accompanying an impaired LVEF has additive adverse implications. Similarly, the diameter and shape of the left ventricle strongly influence prognosis; increased size and ventricular sphericity correlate with excessive mortality. In patients with systolic LV dysfunction, the finding of impaired diastolic relaxation or a restrictive filling pattern (by Doppler echo) is a powerful predictor of 1-year mortality risk.

A severe impairment of objective exercise (functional) capacity, whether measured as maximal exercise capacity (METS or VO_2 max) or submaximal exercise (6-minute walking test distance) is also a strong harbinger of increased annual mortality risk. A patient with a VO_2 max <15 mL/kg/min (4 to 5 METS) has a markedly increased 1-year mortality risk (>20%). In certain patients, the exercise performance trend may be more useful, as the prognostic value of the VO_2 max is limited by the absence of well-defined contemporary 'normal' values adjusted for age and gender in many laboratories. Clinical trial data reveal that a patient with systolic LV dysfunction who cannot walk more than 300 meters in 6 minutes has a substantially greater annual risk of death than one who can walk 450 meters or more.

Other variables indicating a patient at increased morbidity and mortality risk include the presence and severity of atrial and ventricular arrhythmias, a serum sodium <130 mg/dL, and concomitant renal failure. Although not easily or commonly obtained outside of multicenter clinical research trials, neurohormonal markers (norepinephrine, BNP, aldosterone), LV mass, and cardiac histologic findings also yield prognostic information. Table 8 lists the key points examined in this chapter.

Suggested Readings

Alexander M, Grumbach K, Remy L, et al: Congestive heart failure hospitalizations and survival in California: patterns according to race/ethnicity. *Am Heart J* 1999;137:919-927.

Aronow WS, Ahn C, Kronzon I: Prognosis of congestive heart failure in elderly patients with normal versus abnormal left ventricular systolic function associated with coronary artery disease. *Am J Cardiol* 1990;66:1257-1259.

Brater DC, Harris C, Redfern JS, et al: Renal effects of COX-2-selective inhibitors. *Am J Nephrol* 2001;21:1-15.

Cahalin LP, Mathier MA, Semigran MJ, et al: The six-minute walk test predicts peak oxygen uptake and survival in patients with advanced heart failure. *Chest* 1996;110:325-332.

Carson P, Ziesche S, Johnson G, et al: Racial differences in response to therapy for heart failure: analysis of the vasodilator-heart failure trials. Vasodilator-Heart Failure Trial Study Group. *J Card Fail* 1999;5:178-187.

Chatterjee K: Physical examination in heart failure. In: Hosenpud JD, Greenberg BH, eds. *Congestive Heart Failure. Pathophysiology, Diagnosis and Comprehensive Approach to Management*, 2nd ed. Philadelphia, Lippincott Williams and Wilkins, 2000, pp 615-627.

Cheitlin MD, Alpert JS, Armstrong WF, et al: ACC/AHA guidelines for the clinical application of echocardiography. A report of the American College of Cardiology/American Heart Association Task Force on Practice Guidelines (Committee on Clinical Application of Echocardiography). Developed in collaboration with the American Society of Echocardiography. *Circulation* 1997;95:1686-1744.

Chin MH, Goldman L: Gender differences in 1-year survival and quality of life among patients admitted with congestive heart failure. *Med Care* 1998;36:1033-1046.

Connors AF Jr, Speroff T, Dawson NV, et al: The effectiveness of right heart catheterization in the initial care of critically ill patients. SUPPORT Investigators. *JAMA* 1996;276:889-897.

Dao Q, Krishnaswamy P, Kazanegra R, et al: Utility of B-type natriuretic peptide in the diagnosis of congestive heart failure in an urgent-care setting. *J Am Coll Cardiol* 2001;37:379-385.

Davos CH, Doehner W, Rauchhaus M, et al: Obesity and survival in chronic heart failure. *Circulation* 2000;102(suppl I);I-4202.

Drazner MH, Hamilton MA, Fonarow G, et al: Relationship between right and left-sided filling pressures in 1000 patients with advanced heart failure. *J Heart Lung Transplant* 1999;18:1126-1132.

Dries DL, Exner DV, Gersh BJ, et al: Racial differences in the outcome of left ventricular dysfunction [published erratum appears in *N Engl J Med* 1999 Jul 22;341:298]. *N Engl J Med* 1999;340:609-616.

Fuster V, Gersh BJ, Giuliani ER, et al: The natural history of idiopathic dilated cardiomyopathy. *Am J Cardiol* 1981;47:525-531.

Ghali JK, Kadakia S, Cooper RS, et al: Bedside diagnosis of preserved versus impaired left ventricular systolic function in heart failure. *Am J Cardiol* 1991;67:1002-1006.

Gheorghiade M, Bonow RO: Chronic heart failure in the United States: a manifestation of coronary artery disease. *Circulation* 1998;97:282-289.

Hamilton MA, Stevenson LW: Thyroid hormone abnormalities in heart failure: possibilities for therapy. *Thyroid* 1996;6:527-529.

Hermann DD, Greenberg BH: Prognostic factors. In: Poole-Wilson PA, et al, eds. *Heart Failure: Scientific Principles and Clinical Practice.* New York, Churchill Livingstone, 1997, pp 439-454.

Hosenpud JD, Jarcho JA: The cardiomyopathies. In: Hosenpud JD, Greenberg BH, eds. *Congestive Heart Failure. Pathophysiology, Diagnosis and Comprehensive Approach to Management,* 2nd ed. Philadelphia, Lippincott Williams and Wilkins, 2000, pp 281-312.

Hunt SA, Baker DW, Chin MH, et al: ACC/AHA guidelines for the evaluation and management of chronic heart failure in the adult. A report of the American College of Cardiology/American Heart Association Task Force on Practice Guidelines (Committee to Revise the 1995 Guidelines for the Evaluation and Management of Heart Failure). *J Am Coll Cardiol* 2001;38:2101-2113. Full text available at http://www.acc.org/clinical/guidelines/failure/hf_index.htm.

Iriarte M, Murga N, Sagastagoitia D, et al: Congestive heart failure from left ventricular diastolic dysfunction in systemic hypertension. *Am J Cardiol* 1993;71:308-312.

Kannel WB: Epidemiology and prevention of cardiac failure: Framingham Study insights. *Eur Heart J* 1987;8(suppl F):23-26.

Kjekshus J: Arrhythmias and mortality in congestive heart failure. *Am J Cardiol* 1990;65:42I-48I.

Lenihan DJ, Gerson MC, Hoit BD, et al: Mechanisms, diagnosis, and treatment of diastolic heart failure. *Am Heart J* 1995;130:153-166.

Levy D, Larson MG, Vasan RS, et al: The progression from hypertension to congestive heart failure. *JAMA* 1996;275:1557-1562.

Litwin SE, Grossman W: Diastolic dysfunction as a cause of heart failure. *J Am Coll Cardiol* 1993;22:49A-55A.

Maisel A: B-type natriuretic peptide levels: a potential novel "white count" for congestive heart failure. *J Card Fail* 2001;7:183-193.

Massie BM, Shah NB: Evolving trends in the epidemiologic factors of heart failure: rationale for preventive strategies and comprehensive disease management. *Am Heart J* 1997;133:703-712.

Mendes LA, Davidoff R, Cupples LA, et al: Congestive heart failure in patients with coronary artery disease: the gender paradox. *Am Heart J* 1997;134:207-212.

Mortality risk and patterns of practice in 4606 acute care patients with congestive heart failure. The relative importance of age, sex, and medical therapy. Clinical Quality Improvement Network Investigators. *Arch Intern Med* 1996;156:1669-1673.

Nagueh SF: Noninvasive evaluation of hemodynamics by Doppler echocardiography. *Curr Opin Cardiol* 1999;14:217-224.

Nishimura RA, Tajik AJ: Evaluation of diastolic filling of left ventricle in health and disease: Doppler echocardiography is the clinician's Rosetta Stone. *J Am Coll Cardiol* 1997;30:8-18.

Norcross WA, Hermann DD: Heart failure. In: Taylor RB, ed. *Manual of Family Practice*, 2nd ed. Philadelphia, Lippincott Williams and Wilkins, 2002. In press.

Philbin EF, DiSalvo TG: Influence of race and gender on care process, resource use, and hospital-based outcomes in congestive heart failure. *Am J Cardiol* 1998;82:76-81.

Pinamonti B, Zecchin M, Di Lenarda A, et al: Persistence of restrictive left ventricular filling pattern in dilated cardiomyopathy: an ominous prognostic sign. *J Am Coll Cardiol* 1997;29:604-612.

Ritchie JL, Bateman TM, Bonow RO, et al: Guidelines for clinical use of cardiac radionuclide imaging: a report of the American College of Cardiology/American Heart Association Task Force on Assessment of Diagnostic and Therapeutic Cardiovascular Procedures (Committee on Radionuclide Imaging), developed in collaboration with the American Society of Nuclear Cardiology. *J Am Coll Cardiol* 1995;25:521-547.

Shindler DM, Kostis JB, Yusuf S, et al: Diabetes mellitus, a predictor of morbidity and mortality in the Studies of Left Ventricular Dysfunction (SOLVD) Trials and Registry. *Am J Cardiol* 1996;77:1017-1020.

Weber KT, Wilson JR, Janicki JS, et al: Exercise testing in the evaluation of the patient with chronic cardiac failure. *Am Rev Respir Dis* 1984;129:S60-S62.

Wilhelmsen L, Rosengren A, Eriksson H, et al: Heart failure in the general population of men—morbidity, risk factors and prognosis. *J Intern Med* 2001;249:253-261.

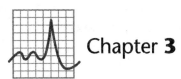 Chapter **3**

Digitalis, Diuretics, and Vasodilator Therapy

A ngiotensin-converting enzyme (ACE) inhibitors and β-blockers are potent neurohormonal modulators that represent the cornerstone of standard medical therapy for heart failure caused by systolic left ventricular dysfunction (LVD). When a patient is clearly intolerant to ACE inhibitors because of refractory cough or allergic reaction, angiotensin-receptor blockers (ARBs) are generally the recommended alternative. This chapter reviews the use of adjunctive agents (digitalis, diuretics) and other alternative vasodilator drugs.

Digoxin
Clinical Trial Indications

Despite more than 2 centuries of use and contemporary outcomes data, digitalis use in chronic heart failure remains controversial and an infrequently prescribed therapy for heart failure in Europe. Sufficient data supporting digoxin (Lanoxin®) utility for symptomatic improvement, including quality of life and exercise duration, resulted in the US Food and Drug Administration's recent approval for its use in mild to moderate heart failure. In addition, the American College of Cardiology/American Heart Association and the

Table 1: Characteristics of Digoxin

- Indicated in NYHA Class II-IV heart failure patients on ACE inhibitors, β-blockers, and diuretics.

- No loading dose necessary in sinus rhythm.

- Dose is 0.125 to 0.250 mg/d depending on age, renal function, and concomitant medications.

- Trough serum concentration 0.8 to 1.2 ng/mL.

NYHA = New York Heart Association

Heart Failure Society of America clinical guidelines recommend digoxin use for symptomatic heart failure patients in the absence of specific contraindications (Table 1). The data used for these decisions included the Digitalis Investigation Group (DIG) mortality trial sponsored by the National Institutes of Health (NIH), along with retrospective analyses from the Prospective Randomized Study of Ventricular Failure and the Efficacy of Digoxin (PROVED) and the Randomized Assessment of the Effect of Digoxin on Inhibitors of the Angiotensin-Converting Enzyme (RADIANCE) trial databases.

The DIG trial was a randomized, double-blind, placebo-controlled mortality trial enrolling nearly 7,800 heart failure patients on background ACE inhibitor and diuretic therapy. Only a small proportion of patients were receiving a β-blocker at study entry, based on trial data available at the time the study was conducted. Most patients (6,800) had heart failure caused by systolic LVD with an ejection fraction (EF) ≤45%. Overall, digitalis administration had a neutral effect on the primary outcome variable of total mortality (35%) after an average follow-up period of approximately 3 years (relative risk ratio [RR] 0.99, P=0.8). Cardiovascular mortality (30%) was also similar in the two groups. Thus, digitalis represents the only available oral agent with mild, positively inotropic activity that does not adversely affect mortality in heart failure populations (Figures 1 and 2).

In the DIG trial, digoxin administration had a beneficial effect on the clinical outcome of heart failure patients for the combined secondary trial end point of hospitalization or need for increased heart failure medication (increased diuretic or ACE inhibitor dose or added therapies). Overall, significantly fewer patients on digoxin (26.8%) than placebo (34.7%) were hospitalized for worsening heart failure (RR 0.72 [95% CI 0.66 to 0.79], $P<0.001$). Further, in a prespecified subgroup analysis of patients with severe heart failure (EF <0.25), a 16% reduction in all-cause mortality or hospitalization was noted for patients receiving digoxin (95% CI 0.07 to 0.24). More notably, heart failure death or hospitalization was reduced by 39% for those patients with severe heart failure who were randomized to digoxin therapy vs placebo (95% CI 0.29 to 0.47).

Digoxin is generally administered to patients with systolic LVD. A subset of 988 patients in the DIG trial had heart failure with a left ventricular ejection fraction (LVEF) >45% but demonstrated similar results to those with systolic LVD. Although it was a small subset, the mortality rate of 23.4% was not altered by digoxin therapy. However, the combined end point of death or hospitalization for worsening heart failure occurred less often in the digoxin-treated group (RR 0.82 [95% CI 0.63 to 1.07]).

Additional evidence showing that digoxin use has additive benefits to ACE inhibitor therapy derives from a contemporary analysis of the combined PROVED and RADIANCE trial databases. When digitalis administration was continued along with an ACE inhibitor and diuretic background therapy, only 4.7% of patients were hospitalized for worsening heart failure. This was significantly less than the 25% of patients on an ACE inhibitor and diuretic combination hospitalized after digoxin withdrawal ($P=0.001$). Hospitalization occurred in 39% of patients withdrawn from digitalis therapy and maintained on diuretic monotherapy

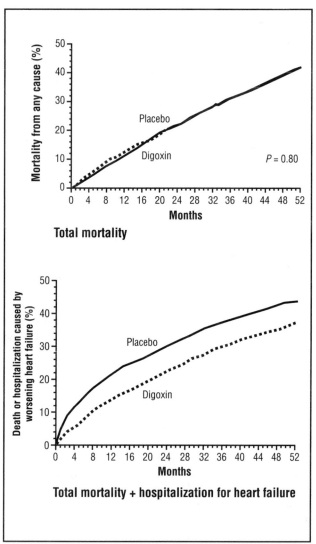

Figure 1: Digitalis Investigation Group (DIG) trial results: primary end point analysis.

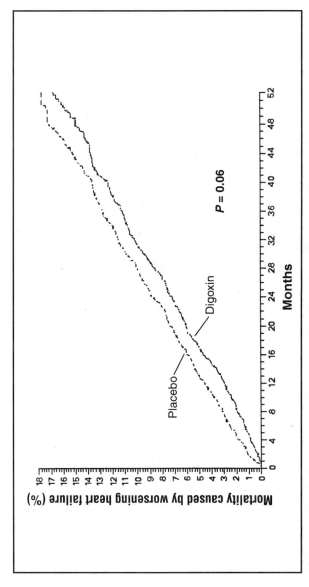

Figure 2: Digitalis Investigation Group (DIG) trial results: secondary end point analysis.

(P <0.001) and in 19% of those continued on digoxin and diuretics but without an ACE inhibitor (P=0.009).

In summary, digoxin use in chronic heart failure is associated with symptomatic improvement, increased exercise tolerance, and clinical stability. Overall, the clinical benefit derived from the use of an inexpensive drug outweighs its risks in most patients who remain symptomatic after ACE inhibitor and diuretic therapy. Whether digoxin administration has incremental benefit when the background therapy consists of an ACE inhibitor, a β-blocker, and diuretics is unknown.

Mechanism of Action

Aside from digoxin's electrophysiologic effects, the traditional perception of digoxin's effect on the cardiovascular system in heart failure is that of a mild positive inotropic agent. This perception is based on the long-known ability of digoxin to inhibit myocardial membrane sodium-potassium adenosine triphosphatase (ATPase) activity (Figure 3). The resultant increase in intracellular calcium concentration through sodium-calcium exchange increases myocardial contractility. Globally, ventricular function (Frank-Starling) curves shift upward and leftward, reflecting increased cardiac work at the same filling pressure. This corresponds to an approximately 5% global increase in LVEF.

Digoxin has also been shown to possess sympathoinhibitory neurohormonal modulating effects, which are probably responsible for its beneficial effects in heart failure. Digoxin reduces heart failure-related autonomic dysfunction by enhancing parasympathetic tone, demonstrated in studies of heart rate variability and peripheral muscle sympathetic nerve activity. Diminished baroreceptor responsiveness is also enhanced by digoxin administration. Reduced baroreceptor reflex activity contributes to enhancement of plasma catecholamine, vasopressin, and renin secretion. Thus, digoxin also acts as a neurohormonal modulator to antagonize sympathetic nervous system hyperactivity.

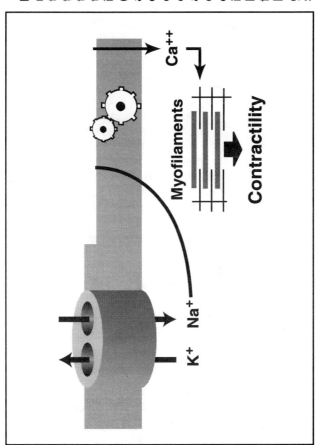

Figure 3: Mechanism of positive inotropic activity of digitalis. Digoxin inhibits the sodium (Na)-potassium (K) adenosine triphosphatase (ATPase), resulting in an increased intracellular sodium concentration. This excess sodium is then available for the sodium-calcium (Ca) exchange. The net increase in intracellular calcium available for myofilament binding results in greater contractile strength.

Clinical Prescription and Monitoring

Although several digitalis glycoside formulations exist, the most widely prescribed form is digoxin (Lanoxin®). Compounds in gel form have 90% to 100% bioavailability, although drugs that increase gastrointestinal motility can reduce absorption, as do binding resins, such as cholestyramine (Questran®) and some antacids. There is no evidence that tachyphylaxis occurs with chronic administration.

For the treatment of chronic heart failure in sinus rhythm, a loading dose is unnecessary. The recommended dose ranges from 0.125 to 0.250 mg/d (Table 1), based on body weight, age, and renal function. Most physicians obtain a serum digoxin concentration (SDC) once steady state is achieved (2 to 3 weeks), as a trough level drawn 6 hours or more after oral dosing. The SDC need not be repeated on a regular basis but should be determined in the setting of worsened renal function, signs or symptoms of digitalis toxicity, or the addition or discontinuation of drugs known to alter the SDC, such as amiodarone, quinidine, spironolactone, and others. Over-the-counter herbal preparations that contain hawthorn berry (*Crataegus*), popular among heart failure patients, have also been reported to elevate the SDC. Hypothyroid patients and those with hypokalemia or hypomagnesemia are more susceptible to digoxin toxicity. Whether an ideal 'therapeutic' SDC exists is controversial. Most heart failure experts recommend a trough SDC between 0.8 and 1.2 ng/mL, the levels achieved in the DIG and RADIANCE trials, respectively. Loading doses are unnecessary in the chronic heart failure patient. The pharmacodynamic properties of digitalis are shown in Table 2.

The effects of digoxin on the resting electrocardiogram (EKG) are well described. Although digoxin toxicity is a clinical diagnosis, it typically manifests as either excitatory (supraventricular tachycardia with block or ventricular extrasystoles, tachycardia, or fibrillation) or suppressant rhythm disturbances (sinus bradycardia, sinoatrial or

Table 2: Pharmacodynamic Properties of Digitalis

Oral absorption	60% to 75%
Protein binding	25%
Volume of distribution	6 (3-9) L/kg
Half-life	36 (26-46) h
Elimination	Renal
Onset	
IV	5-30 min
oral	30-90 min
Maximal effect	
IV	2-4 h
oral	3-6 h
Duration	2-6 d
Suggested level	0.8-1.2 ng/mL

atrioventricular block). The noncardiac manifestations of digitalis toxicity are shown in Table 3.

Diuretics

There are no clinical trial data prospectively evaluating the overall impact of diuretic therapy on mortality in the heart failure patient population. Clearly, diuretics are useful and necessary adjuncts to medical therapy for congestive heart failure (CHF) symptoms caused by sodium and water retention, but they do not maintain clinical stability when used as monotherapy. However, while diuretics promote renal sodium and water excretion, they activate the renin-angiotensin-aldosterone axis, potentiate hypotensive effects of ACE inhibitors, and may decrease cardiac output

Table 3: Noncardiac Manifestations of Digitalis Toxicity

Gastrointestinal
- Nausea
- Vomiting
- Diarrhea

Nervous System
- Depression
- Disorientation
- Paresthesias

Visual
- Blurred vision
- Scotomas
- Yellow-green vision

Hyperestrogenism
- Gynecomastia
- Galactorrhea

if overused, especially in patients with diastolic LVD. Generally, diuretics create electrolyte wasting and attributable side effects. Diuretic prescriptions should generally be accompanied by a recommendation for a dietary sodium restriction of 2,000 to 3,000 mg/d for the typical patient with heart failure. Fluid restriction is best reserved for the patient with excessive oral fluid intake, symptomatic hyponatremia, or diuretic refractoriness.

Diuretics should be used for congestive symptoms or signs and titrated according to an estimated 'dry' weight, which is based on optimal filling pressures and symptoms, without exacerbating symptomatic hypotension. Underuse of diuretic therapy is common, but excessive diuresis-limiting ventricular preload may, in turn, limit the (blood pressure) tolerance to oral vasodilator titration. Appropriate use of diuretic therapy is a key element in heart failure pharmacology. Intensification of diuretic and/or vasodilator therapy may be accompanied by a modest elevation and plateau in blood urea nitrogen and serum creatinine concentration. While often troubling to physicians, this finding is typically 'physiologic' and not considered indicative of intrinsic or irreversible renal dysfunction. Mild to moderate azotemia warrants a review of the patient's medication profile to avoid concomitant administration of nephrotoxic drugs (ie, nonsteroidal anti-inflammatory drugs [NSAIDs]) and to determine if dose reduction in medications dependent on renal clearance (ie, digoxin) is warranted. It is essential, however, to recognize progressive renal insufficiency caused by decreasing renal perfusion, which can result from a decline in cardiac output, renovascular disease, excessive vasodilation (shunting), or hypotension.

The site of action of the various diuretic agents is shown in Figure 4. Generally, the most potent and widely used diuretic agents for heart failure management are the loop of Henle-active agents.

Loop Diuretics

Drugs acting upon the ascending limb of the renal medullary loop of Henle are considered the agents of choice for the treatment of heart failure (Table 4). They are actively secreted in the proximal renal tubule and, therefore, depend on glomerular filtration to reach their site of action. Each drug has a maximum fractional excretion of filtered sodium (FeNa) of 20% to 25%, reflecting increased potency when compared with an FeNa of only 5% to 10% for the thiazide group.

Diuretic efficacy depends on the peak serum concentration reaching the renal glomeruli. Heart failure can affect drug pharmacokinetics in several ways. Delayed absorption caused by gut edema from high central venous pressure can reduce the peak serum concentration. The volume of distribution is also variable in the setting of chronic heart failure. Further, relative hypotension or reduced cardiac output that produces a limitation in renal blood flow reduces the glomerular filtration rate (GFR). A summary of the loop diuretic mechanism of action and adverse reactions can be found in Table 5.

Generally, the limitations of loop diuretics can be overcome by successively increasing the administered dose. The

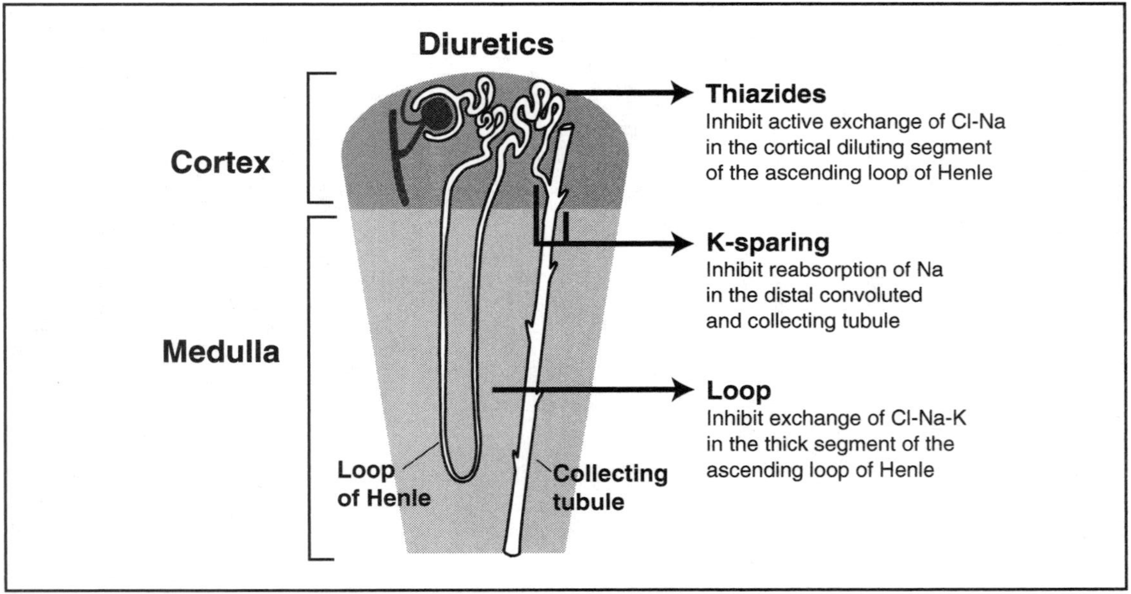

Figure 4: Site of action of diuretic agents on the nephron.

onset of action with intravenous (IV) administration is within minutes, making this route of administration preferable for the acutely symptomatic or hospitalized patient. Some physicians have a strong preference for loop diuretic administration by continuous infusion, although the efficacy of this approach is controversial. For the patient with profound fluid overload, continuous infusion of a loop diuretic can result in a 'steady-state' diuresis, along with a more predictable rate of electrolyte loss that requires replacement. Similarly, some evidence shows that bumetanide (Bumex®) has greater efficacy than furosemide (Lasix®) in the setting of markedly reduced glomerular filtration, probably caused by proximal tubular filtration when secretion is limited. A continuous infusion of furosemide (>0.5 mg/kg/24 h) or bumetanide (>0.125 mg/kg/24 h) has been shown to augment diuresis without excessive electrolyte loss. Inadequate diuresis and failure to assess the efficacy of oral diuretic administration before hospital discharge are common management errors leading to rapid symptomatic relapse and readmission.

In addition to electrolyte abnormalities and contraction alkalosis, loop diuretics have several other side effects. With rapid IV administration of high-dose loop diuretics, hearing loss to the point of deafness can result from middle-ear toxicity. Skin reactions, from photosensitivity to rashes, are not uncommon, and hypersensitivity reactions can also manifest as interstitial nephritis. High doses of loop diuretics can worsen hyperglycemia and carbohydrate intolerance. Perhaps the most unpleasant and perplexing side effects of loop diuretics for patients with chronic heart failure are hyperuricemia and gout, which are caused by uric acid reabsorption.

Thiazide Diuretics

Thiazide diuretics inhibit sodium reabsorption in the distal renal tubule. They are generally not useful as diuretic monotherapy in heart failure and are ineffective when the GFR falls below 30 mL/min. In addition, to achieve a volume diuresis equivalent to that with loop diuretics, thiazides produce greater potassium wasting.

69

Table 4: Commonly Used Diuretic Agents

Agent	Form	Dose Range	Maximum Daily Total Dose
Loop diuretics			
furosemide (Lasix®)	IV	10-200 mg	200 mg
	PO	20-200 mg b.i.d.	400 mg
bumetanide (Bumex®)	IV	0.5-2 mg	8 mg
	PO	1.0-4 mg b.i.d.	8 mg
torsemide (Demadex®)	IV	20-100 mg	100 mg
	PO	10-120 mg q.d.	200 mg
ethacrynic acid (Edecrin®)	No longer manufactured in United States		
Thiazide diuretics			

Duration of Action	Comment
	Generally effective diuretic mono-therapy in heart failure. Inhibit active NaCl transport in medullary ascending limb of the loop of Henle. Potassium and magnesium loss may require replacement.
~2-4 h	↓ efficacy with CrCl < 30.
~6-8 h	↓↓ absorption in systemic venous congestion.
~2-4 h	Retains efficacy when CrCl < 30 or if azotemia is present.
~6-8 h	↓ absorption with systemic venous congestion.
~3-6 h	
~6-12 h	Near 100% oral bioavailability.
	Only loop diuretic without a sulfhydryl group for sulfa-allergic patients.
	Generally not effective as mono-therapy in moderate to severe heart failure. Act on distal convoluted tubule and cortical ascending limb of the loop of Henle.

(continued on next page.)

Table 4: Commonly Used Diuretic Agents
(continued)

Agent	Form	Dose Range	Maximum Daily Total Dose
Thiazide diuretics *(continued)*			
chlorothiazide (Diuril®)	IV	250-500 mg b.i.d.	1,000 mg
	PO	250-500 mg b.i.d.	1,000 mg
hydrochlorothiazide (Lotensin®, Vaseretic®, Zestoretic®)	PO	25-50 mg q.d.	100 mg
metolazone (Zaroxolyn®, Mykrox®)	PO	2.5-5.0 mg b.i.d.	10 mg
Potassium-sparing diuretics			
amiloride (Midamor®)	PO	5-20 mg q.d.	20 mg
triamterene (Dyazide®, Maxzide®)	PO	100 mg b.i.d	200 mg
spironolactone (Aldactone®)	PO	12.5-200 mg q.d. to t.i.d.	400 mg

PO = oral; IV = intravenous; q.d. = daily
b.i.d. = twice daily; q.o.d. = alternating days
CrCl = creatinine clearance
NYHA = New York Heart Association

Duration of Action	Comment
~2-4 h	Used as adjunct to potentiate loop diuretic efficacy when higher doses of the former are required, with marked increase in electrolyte loss.
~6-8 h	
~6-12 h	
~8-24 h	
	Generally not used as monotherapy in heart failure. Helpful in patients with potassium wasting on loop diuretics. Frequent monitoring for hyperkalemia is advisable.
18-24 h	
~8 h	Do not combine with furosemide (prevents furosemide secretion).
8-24 h	Recommended for use in NYHA Class III-IV at 12.5-25 mg q.d. or q.o.d. for neurohormonal modulation. Monitor serum potassium closely.

Table 5: Loop Diuretics

Mechanism of Action

- Excrete 15% to 25% of proximally filtered sodium load, dose dependent
- Increase potassium, magnesium, and calcium excretion
- Increase renal prostaglandin release via renal afferent vasodilation

Adverse Reactions

- Electrolyte disturbances
- Metabolic alkalosis
- Metabolic disturbances: hyperuricemia, hyperglycemia, lipid effects
- Azotemia
- Orthostasis
- Rapid IV infusion causes irreversible ototoxicity and deafness
- Hypotension
- Rash
- Sun sensitivity

Metolazone (Zaroxolyn®) is particularly potent in this regard, acting in concert on both proximal and distal tubules. Thiazide diuretics share most of the side effects seen with loop diuretics, although an association with pancreatitis appears be unique to this drug category (Tables 4 and 6).

Thiazide diuretics can be used in combination with loop diuretics to augment natriuresis when the dose of the loop diuretic is near maximum. Diuretic resistance is partly related to chronic loop diuretic administration, typically at escalating doses. Chronic exposure results in progressive hypertrophy of distal renal tubular en-

Table 6: Thiazide Diuretics

Mechanism of Action
- Excrete 5% to 10% of filtered sodium load
- No dose response
- Increase in potassium, calcium, and magnesium loss greater than with loop diuretics
- Induce renal vasoconstriction
- Increase uric acid excretion

Adverse Reactions
- Electrolyte disturbances
- Metabolic alkalosis
- Metabolic disturbances: hyperglycemia, lipid effects, pancreatitis
- Azotemia
- Orthostasis
- Hypotension
- Rash
- Sun sensitivity

dothelial cells, which reabsorb sodium more avidly. By combining a thiazide diuretic with a loop-active drug, this compensatory hypertrophy can be overridden. The cost, however, is significant electrolyte loss. Therefore, the combination should primarily be used for patients refractory to high-dose loop diuretics.

Potassium-Sparing Diuretics

Potassium (K)-sparing diuretics are used infrequently for direct diuretic activity, which is quite mild. Several are formulated in combination with thiazides for the treatment of hypertension, but they are generally not useful in heart failure. For patients with excessive potassium loss on loop diuretics, coincident administration of these agents can be helpful.

The use of spironolactone (Aldactone®) at a low dose (12.5 to 25 mg/d) as a systemic neurohormonal (aldosterone) antagonist for New York Heart Association (NYHA) Class III and IV patients is reviewed in Chapter 4. When spironolactone is used even in small doses, care must be taken to monitor frequently for the development of hyperkalemia, particularly in patients with preexisting renal insufficiency (serum creatinine >2.4 mg/dL) or with renal tubular acidosis. Between 10% and 15% of patients on chronic spironolactone therapy develop painful gynecomastia, which resolves upon discontinuation (Tables 4 and 7).

Alternative or Additional Vasodilator Therapy

The treatment paradigm for heart failure that preceded the current neurohormonal model used systemic vasodilators to reduce ventricular preload and systemic vascular resistance, thereby indirectly improving cardiac output and central hemodynamics without direct inotropic stimulation. Patients with chronic heart failure often benefit from the addition of a vasodilator to standard medical therapy, particularly when blood pressure remains relatively preserved. Other patients may be unable to tolerate ACE inhibition because of rash, intractable cough, or angioedema.

The influence of venous and arterial vasodilator therapy on cardiac output and ventricular filling pressures in a failing ventricle with reduced contractility is illustrated in Figure 5. Arterial vasodilation increases cardiac output while reducing LV end-diastolic pressure; venodilation reduces filling pressures (symptoms) with minimal effect on cardiac output. ACE inhibitor therapy as a neurohormonal antagonist with vasodilatory activity derived from positive results in early comparative vasodilator trials. ACE inhibitors and ARBs are compared in Chapter 4. This section reviews non-ACE, non-ARB vasodilators as addi-

Table 7: Potassium-Sparing Diuretics

Mechanism of Action

- Excrete <5% of proximally filtered sodium load, dose dependent
- Inhibit exchange of sodium, thus retaining hydrogen or potassium
- Spironolactone is a direct aldosterone receptor antagonist

Adverse Reactions

- Electrolyte disturbances
- Metabolic acidosis
- Hyperkalemia
- Hyponatremia
- Muscle cramps
- Weakness
- Rash
- Pruritus
- 10% to 15% incidence of painful gynecomastia with spironolactone

tional or alternative therapy to ACE inhibitors in chronic heart failure.

Hydralazine and Nitrate Combinations

The initial Vasodilator Heart Failure Trial (V-HeFT) was the first randomized, placebo-controlled trial to add a vasodilator (combined hydralazine/isosorbide dinitrate [Hyd/Iso] or prazosin [Minipress®]) to the medical regimen of patients with heart failure and symptomatic systolic LVD. At the time, the trial was considered large, with 642 patients predominantly in NYHA Classes III and IV. The combined venous and arteriolar vasodilator com-

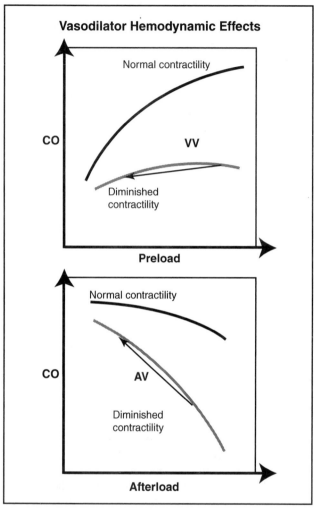

Figure 5: The influence of vasodilator therapy on hemodynamics in the setting of impaired LV function. CO = cardiac output; VV = venous vasodilator; AV = arterial vasodilator.

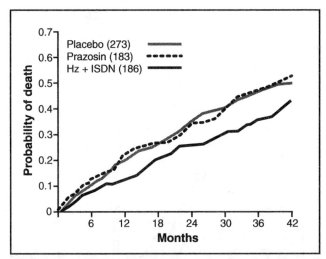

Figure 6: V-HeFT I trial results evaluating the effect of vasodilator therapy on survival in chronic symptomatic heart failure. Hz = hydralazine; ISDN = isosorbide dinitrate.

bination had a significantly favorable effect on survival compared with either placebo or prazosin (Figure 6). Mortality was reduced by 23% with Hyd/Iso, while the α-blocker provided no advantage over placebo, with a 1-year mortality risk of approximately 20%.

V-HeFT II compared the relative efficacy of Hyd/Iso to that of enalapril (Vaseretic®) in reducing mortality in 804 men with chronic heart failure and an LVEF <0.45. The target doses were: hydralazine 75 mg q.i.d., isosorbide dinitrate 40 q.i.d. (with a 10-hour drug-free interval at night), and enalapril 10 mg b.i.d. Two-year mortality was lower in the enalapril group (18% vs 25%, P=0.016), and this difference persisted throughout the 5-year follow-up period. The Hyd/Iso arm of V-HeFT II confirmed the findings of V-HeFT, with an annual mortality risk of 13% on active therapy (Figure 7). Interestingly, while enalapril therapy improved sur-

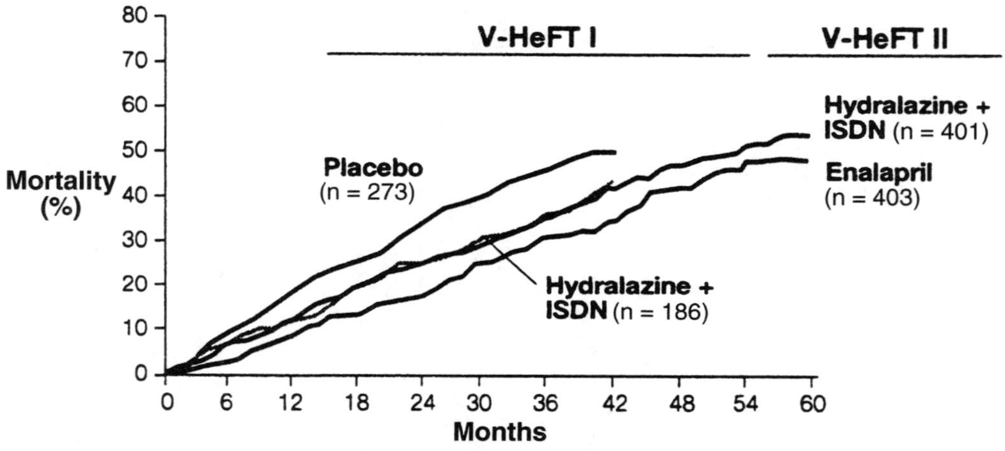

Risk reduction at 2 years **V-HeFT I** = 34% (*P* = .028) **V-HeFT II** = 28% (*P* = .016)

Cohn et al. *N Engl J Med* 1986;314;1547-1552. Cohn et al. *N Engl J Med* 1991;325;303-310.

Figure 7: V-HeFT I and II: effects of hydralazine/isosorbide dinitrate in heart failure.

vival to a greater degree (9% annually), the Hyd/Iso group had greater improvements in exercise capacity and LVEF.

For patients with significant renal insufficiency precluding the use of ACE inhibitors or ARBs, the combination of Hyd/Iso is an effective alternative therapy because it tends to increase renal cortical blood flow. While the hemodynamic effects of hydralazine in heart failure have been extensively studied, hydralazine has not been evaluated as monotherapy in heart failure mortality trials. Administration yields a reduction in systemic and pulmonary vascular resistance that augments stroke volume and cardiac output. The 5% to 10% reduction in mean arterial pressure results from a greater reduction in diastolic vs systolic pressure. While vasodilation is hemodynamically advantageous, it produces a reflex tachycardia that stimulates the sympathetic nervous system and increases renin activity in plasma (presumably as a result of increased secretion of renin by the renal juxtaglomerular cells in response to reflex sympathetic discharge). Heightened renin-angiotensin-aldosterone and sympathetic nervous system tone are considered disadvantageous in chronic heart failure. The side effect and dosing profiles of hydralazine can be found in Table 8.

Similarly, the independent effect of nitrates on survival in chronic heart failure is unknown. Isosorbide dinitrate was the active agent responsible for the improvement in exercise tolerance noted in the V-HeFT trials. However, its use does not result in a sustained increase in systemic catecholamines. These agents facilitate improvement in peripheral vasodilator capacity, and nitrate administration helps restore endothelial endogenous nitric oxide synthase function by serving as a source of nitric oxide. Nitrates are useful as adjunctive therapy for symptomatic relief in patients with heart failure caused by underlying ischemic heart disease, those with subendocardial ischemia caused by increased wall stress, and those with moderate pulmonary hypertension. Nitrates reduce the effective mitral

Table 8: Hydralazine*

Side Effect Profile
Common
- Headache, anorexia, vomiting, diarrhea, palpitations, tachycardia, angina pectoris

Less Frequent
- *Digestive:* constipation, paralytic ileus
- *Cardiovascular:* hypotension, paradoxical pressor response, edema
- *Respiratory:* dyspnea
- *Neurologic:* peripheral neuritis, evidenced by paresthesia, numbness, and tingling; dizziness; tremors; muscle cramps; psychotic reactions characterized by depression, disorientation, or anxiety
- *Genitourinary:* difficulty urinating
- *Hematologic:* blood dyscrasias, consisting of reduction in hemoglobin and red cell count, leukopenia, agranulocytosis, purpura, lymphadenopathy, splenomegaly

regurgitant orifice area and seem to improve ventricular diastolic function as well. Avoidance of pharmacodynamic tolerance can be easily accomplished by scheduling nitrate-free intervals. The administration of hydralazine in combination with isosorbide dinitrate (Hyd/Iso) also seems to minimize the development of nitrate tolerance. Nitrate formulations are available in sustained-release forms, as well as in the mononitrate formulation, which is a primary metabolite of isosorbide dinitrate. The side effect profile of isosorbide can be found in Table 9.

Less Frequent *(continued)*

- *Hypersensitivity:* rash, urticaria, pruritus, fever, arthralgia, eosinophilia, and, rarely, hepatitis
- *Other:* nasal congestion, flushing; lacrimation, conjunctivitis

Heart Failure Dosing
- *Available dosages:* 10-mg, 25-mg, 50-mg, and 100-mg tablets
- *Dose interval:* t.i.d. to q.i.d.
- *Total daily dose range:* 40 to 300 mg
- *Peak effect:* 1 to 2 h
- *Half-life:* 3 to 7 h

* Hydralazine is subject to polymorphic acetylation; slow acetylators generally have higher plasma levels of hydralazine and require or tolerate lower doses.

Calcium-Channel Blockers

First-generation calcium-channel blockers (CCBs) are not recommended for use in heart failure because of systolic ventricular dysfunction caused by myocardial depressant (negative inotropic) effects. Newer dihydropyridine CCB drugs, such as amlodipine (Norvasc®) and felodipine (Plendil®), have greater vasoselectivity (fewer myocardial depressant effects) and have been studied in heart failure populations. They appear to have neutral effects on patient neurohormonal profile. However, their use has appeal for the treatment of angina or residual hypertension

Table 9: Isosorbide Dinitrate

Side Effect Profile

Common
- Headache may be severe and persistent

Less Common
- Cutaneous vasodilation with flushing
- Lightheadedness, dizziness, and weakness
- Hypotension may be accompanied by paradoxical bradycardia
- Additive effect to alcohol
- Marked additive and potentially fatal hypotension if combined with sildenafil (Viagra®)

Extremely Rare
- Methemoglobinemia
- Allergic reaction

Heart Failure Dosing
- Available dosages: 5-mg, 10-mg, 20-mg, 30-mg, and 40-mg tablets
- Dose interval: b.i.d. to q.i.d. (t.i.d. typical with 8 or more hours of nitrate-free interval)
- Daily dose: 30 to 480 mg
- Average bioavailability: approximately 25%

in patients on standard heart failure therapy who are intolerant of or who have strong contraindications to β-blockade. Patients with heart failure and preserved systolic function and/or LV hypertrophy may also derive symptomatic benefit from CCB therapy; however, no morbidity or mortality data exist to guide agent selection at this time. The peripheral vasodilatation induced by CCBs has the common side effect of peripheral edema, which may represent a confusing physical finding when evaluating signs of heart failure in individual patients.

V-HeFT III examined the effects of felodipine on exercise capacity and survival in chronic heart failure as additive therapy to ACE inhibitors, digoxin, and diuretics (Figure 8). Felodipine treatment had no effect on mortality in this population, although there was a worrying trend toward an adverse outcome as the study progressed. There was also no benefit observed in exercise tolerance from active CCB therapy.

Amlodipine was evaluated in the Prospective Randomized Amlodipine Survival Evaluation (PRAISE) trials, which added amlodipine or placebo to background heart failure therapy of an ACE inhibitor, digoxin, and diuretics. Although, overall, the trial demonstrated a neutral effect on survival, a retrospective subset analysis detected a significant improvement in survival in nonischemic heart failure patients. PRAISE-2 was conducted to further assess and validate this possibility in a population of patients with nonischemic cardiomyopathy and symptomatic heart failure. When evaluated prospectively, there was no survival advantage (or disadvantage) attributable to amlodipine administration in this population.

Summary

Digoxin, diuretics, and vasodilators are useful adjuncts to the standard medical therapy for chronic heart failure caused by systolic ventricular dysfunction. Diuretics are necessary in most, but not all, patients with heart failure for control of congestive symptoms caused by avid sodium and water retention. Available data from clinical trials demonstrate that digoxin, felodipine, and amlodipine have neutral effects on total mortality when added to a background regimen that includes an ACE inhibitor and diuretic.

Digoxin provides an outcome benefit of clinical stability (decreased hospitalization for worsening heart failure) and

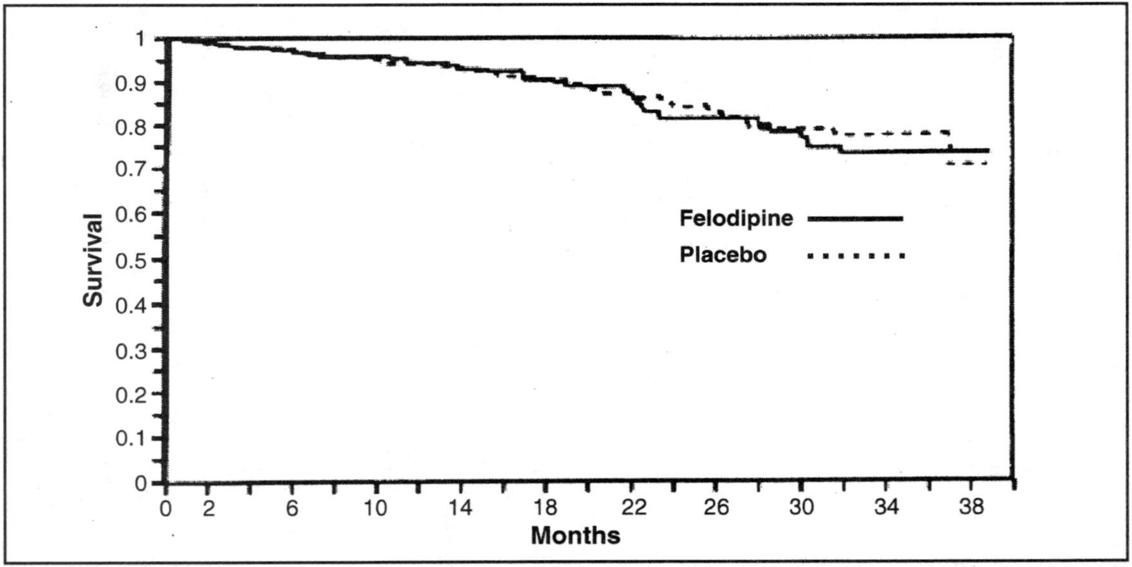

Figure 8: V-HeFT III trial data. Comparison of survival in heart failure patients on felodipine and placebo. Background ACE inhibitor therapy.

is relatively inexpensive. Amlodipine or felodipine may be considered for use in the heart failure patient with residual hypertension or angina despite baseline medical therapy. For patients unable to tolerate ACE inhibitors or ARBs, amlodipine or felodipine may be used as well, although placebo-controlled mortality data support the more cumbersome combination of hydralazine and nitrates in patients with systolic LV dysfunction who are not on ACE inhibitors. Additive nitrate therapy may also be considered for the symptomatic patient with underlying ischemic heart disease, diastolic dysfunction, or mitral regurgitation. Nitrates are generally safe and effective in improving exercise capacity. β-Blockers have recently been added to ACE inhibitor therapy as a vital component of standard care for heart failure and systolic dysfunction. The incremental benefit of these drugs when added to a medical regimen including a β-blocker is unknown.

Suggested Readings

Aaser E, Gullestad L, Tollofsrud S, et al: Effect of bolus injection versus continuous infusion of furosemide on diuresis and neurohormonal activation in patients with severe congestive heart failure. *Scand J Clin Lab Invest* 1997;57:361-367.

Abrams J: Beneficial actions of nitrates in cardiovascular disease. *Am J Cardiol* 1996;77:31C-37C.

Bayliss J, Norell M, Canepa-Anson R, et al: Untreated heart failure: clinical and neuroendocrine effects of introducing diuretics. *Br Heart J* 1987;57:17-22.

Brater DC: Diuretic therapy. *N Engl J Med* 1998;339:387-395.

Brater DC, Harris C, Redfern JS, et al: Renal effects of COX-2-selective inhibitors. *Am J Nephrol* 2001;21:1-15.

Cody RJ, Covit AB, Schaer GL, et al: Sodium and water balance in chronic congestive heart failure. *J Clin Invest* 1986;77:1441-1452.

Cody RJ, Kubo SH, Pickworth KK: Diuretic treatment for the sodium retention of congestive heart failure. *Arch Intern Med* 1994;154:1905-1914.

Cohn JN, Archibald DG, Ziesche S, et al: Effect of vasodilator therapy on mortality in chronic congestive heart failure. Results of a Veterans Administration Cooperative Study. *N Engl J Med* 1986;314:1547-1552.

Cohn JN, Johnson G, Ziesche S, et al: A comparison of enalapril with hydralazine-isosorbide dinitrate in the treatment of chronic congestive heart failure. *N Engl J Med* 1991;325:303-310.

Cohn JN, Ziesche S, Smith R, et al: Effect of the calcium antagonist felodipine as supplementary vasodilator therapy in patients with chronic heart failure treated with enalapril: V-HeFT III. Vasodilator-Heart Failure Trial (V-HeFT) Study Group. *Circulation* 1997;96:856-863.

Dormans TP, Gerlad PG, Russell FG, et al: Combination diuretic therapy in severe congestive heart failure. *Drugs* 1998;55:165-172.

Ellison DH: The physiologic basis of diuretic synergism: its role in treating diuretic resistance. *Ann Intern Med* 1991;114:886-894.

Epstein M, Lepp BA, Hoffman DS, et al: Potentiation of furosemide by metolazone in refractory edema. *Curr Ther Res Clin Exp* 1977;21:656-667.

Gheorghiade M, Ferguson D: Digoxin. A neurohormonal modulator in heart failure? *Circulation* 1991;84:2181-2186.

Gheorghiade M, Hall VB, Jacobsen G, et al: Effects of increasing maintenance dose of digoxin on left ventricular function and neurohormones in patients with chronic heart failure treated with diuretics and angiotensin-converting enzyme inhibitors. *Circulation* 1995;92:1801-1807.

Gogia H, Mehra A, Parikh S, et al: Prevention of tolerance to hemodynamic effects of nitrates with concomitant use of hydralazine in patients with chronic heart failure. *J Am Coll Cardiol* 1995;26:1575-1580.

Goldstein RE, Boccuzzi SJ, Cruess D, et al: Diltiazem increases late-onset congestive heart failure in postinfarction patients with early reduction in ejection fraction. The Adverse Experience Committee; and the Multicenter Diltiazem Postinfarction Research Group. *Circulation* 1991;83:52-60.

Heart Failure Society of America Committee Members and Executive Council: Heart Failure Society of America (HFSA) practice guidelines. HFSA guidelines for the management of patients with heart failure due to left ventricular systolic dysfunction—pharmacological approaches. *Heart Fail* 2000;6:1.

Hermann DD: Naturoceutical agents and cardiovascular medicine—the hope, hype and the harm. *ACC Current Journal Review* 1999;8:53-57.

Hermann DD, Greenberg BH: Refractory heart failure: beyond standard therapy. In: Sharpe N, ed. *Heart Failure Management.* London, Martin Dunitz, 2000, vol 15, pp 199-216.

Hunt SA, Baker DW, Chin MH, et al: ACC/AHA guidelines for the evaluation and management of chronic heart failure in the adult. A report of the American College of Cardiology/American Heart Association Task Force on Practice Guidelines (Committee to Revise the 1995 Guidelines for the Evaluation and Management of Heart Failure). *J Am Coll Cardiol* 2001;38:2101-2113. Full text available at http://www.acc.org/clinical/guidelines/failure/hf_index.htm.

Lee DC, Johnson RA, Bingham JB, et al: Heart failure in outpatients: a randomized trial of digoxin versus placebo. *N Engl J Med* 1982;306:699-705.

Leier CV, Dei Cas L, Metra M: Clinical relevance and management of the major electrolyte abnormalities in congestive heart failure: hyponatremia, hypokalemia and hypomagnesemia. *Am Heart J* 1994:128:564-574.

Massie B, Chatterjee K, Werner J, et al: Hemodynamic advantage of combined administration of hydralazine orally and nitrates nonparenterally in the vasodilator therapy of chronic heart failure. *Am J Cardiol* 1977;40:794-801.

Murray MD, Forthofer MM, Bennett SK, et al: Effectiveness of torsemide and furosemide in the treatment of congestive heart failure: results of a prospective, randomized trial [abstract]. *Circulation* 1999;100(suppl 1):300.

Packer M: Calcium channel blockers in chronic heart failure. The risks of "physiologically rational" therapy [editorial]. *Circulation* 1990;82:2254-2257.

Packer M, Gottlieb SS, Kessler PD: Hormone-electrolyte interactions in the pathogenesis of lethal cardiac arrhythmias in patients with congestive heart failure. Basis of a new physiologic approach to control of arrhythmia. *Am J Med* 1986;80:23-29.

Packer M, Lee WH, Medina N, et al: Functional renal insufficiency during long-term therapy with captopril and enalapril in severe chronic heart failure. *Ann Intern Med* 1987;106:346-354.

Packer M, O'Connor CM, Ghali JK, et al: Effect of amlodipine on morbidity and mortality in severe chronic heart failure. Prospective Randomized Amlodipine Survival Evaluation Study Group. *N Engl J Med* 1996;335:1107-1114.

Parker M, Gheorghiade M, Young JB, et al: Withdrawal of digoxin from patients with chronic heart failure treated with angiotensin-converting enzyme inhibitors. RADIANCE Study. *N Engl J Med* 1993;329:1-7.

Patterson JH, Adams KF Jr, Applefeld MM, et al: Oral torsemide in patients with chronic congestive heart failure: effects on body weight, edema, and electrolyte excretion. Torsemide Investigators Group. *Pharmacotherapy* 1994;14:514-521.

Pierpont GL, Cohn JN, Franciosa JA: Combined oral hydralazine-nitrate therapy in left ventricular failure. Hemodynamic equivalency to sodium nitroprusside. *Chest* 1978;73:8-13.

Pitt B, Zannad F, Remme WJ, et al: The effect of spironolactone on morbidity and mortality in patients with severe heart failure. Randomized Aldactone Evaluation Study Investigators. *N Engl J Med* 1999;341:709-717.

Risler T, Schwab A, Kramer B, et al: Comparative pharmacokinetics and pharmacodynamics of loop diuretics in renal failure. *Cardiology* 1994;84(suppl 2):155-161.

Rude RK: Physiology of magnesium metabolism and the important role of magnesium in potassium deficiency. *Am J Cardiol* 1989;63:31G-34G.

Sica DA, Deedwania P: Pharmacotherapy in congestive heart failure. Principles of combination diuretic therapy in congestive heart failure. *Congest Heart Fail* 1997;3:29-38.

Sica DA, Gehr TW: Diuretic combinations in refractory oedema states: pharmacokinetic-pharmacodynamic relationships. *Clin Pharmacokinet* 1996;30:229-249.

Steiness E, Olesen KH: Cardiac arrhythmias induced by hypokalaemia and potassium loss during maintenance digoxin therapy. *Br Heart J* 1976;38:167-172.

Stevenson LW, Massie BM, Francis GS: Optimizing therapy for complex or refractory heart failure: a management algorithm. *Am Heart J* 1998;135:S293-S309.

Tan LB, Murray RG, Littler WA: Felodipine in patients with chronic heart failure: discrepant haemodynamic and clinical effects. *Br Heart J* 1987;58:122-128.

The effect of digoxin on mortality and morbidity in patients with heart failure. The Digitalis Investigation Group. *N Engl J Med* 1997;336:525-533.

Uretsky BF, Young JB, Shahidi FE, et al: Randomized study assessing the effect of digoxin withdrawal in patients with mild to moderate chronic congestive heart failure: results of the PROVED trial. PROVED Investigative Group. *J Am Coll Cardiol* 1993;22:955-962.

Wilson JR, Reichek N, Dunkman WB, et al: Effect of diuresis on the performance of the failing left ventricle in man. *Am J Med* 1981;70:234-239.

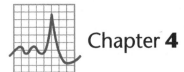

Chapter **4**

Drugs That Block the Renin-Angiotensin-Aldosterone System to Prevent and Treat Heart Failure

For more than 3 decades, a basic tenet of the pathogenesis of heart failure has been that the renin-angiotensin system (RAS) plays an important role in its development. What is perhaps most interesting (and somewhat unexpected) is that our understanding of the role of the RAS in the development of heart failure has steadily expanded over time, and further insights continue to be revealed. Initially, RAS activation was believed to influence the development and progression of heart failure by hemodynamic effects alone. However, convincing evidence now shows that the RAS promotes cardiac remodeling, a process critical to the progressive worsening in systolic and diastolic function, which ultimately results in heart failure.

There is also more recent evidence demonstrating that the impact of the RAS on the heart may be considerably broader in scope than was initially realized, including the role of the RAS in conditions such as hypertension, left ventricular hypertrophy (LVH), coronary artery atherosclerosis, progressive renal dysfunction, and coronary thrombosis. All of these are related to the development of cardiac dysfunction or manifestations of heart failure. Not surprisingly, drugs that block the RAS have assumed a central role in the management of patients with overt heart failure or who are at risk for developing this condition in the future. Thus, an understanding of the role of the RAS in the pathogenesis of heart failure and the appropriate settings for initiation of treatment are essential to providing optimal therapy.

The RAS: A Tale of Two Systems

Angiotensin II (Ang II), the main effector molecule of the RAS, is generated from its precursor molecule, angiotensinogen, through the sequential cleavage of amino acids by a series of proteolytic enzymes. Angiotensinogen is initially altered by renin activity, with the resultant formation of Ang I. This inactive peptide is, in turn, a substrate for angiotensin-converting enzyme (ACE), which cleaves further amino acids from Ang I and generates Ang II. The physiologic and pathophysiologic effects of Ang II occur when it interacts with specific cell surface receptors. An overview of this process is shown in Figure 1. Two major classes of angiotensin receptors have been identified.[1] The type 1 Ang II (AT_1) receptor has seven transmembrane domains, a structure that is associated with cell growth. Virtually all Ang II effects associated with heart failure, such as arterial vasoconstriction, salt and water retention, and growth of cells in cardiovascular and renal tissue, are mediated by the AT_1 receptor. A second class of Ang II receptor, the type 2 (AT_2), has been identified in human subjects and other species.[1-4] Although some evidence shows that the AT_2 receptor may have effects on blood pressure and cell growth opposite those associated with the AT_1 receptor,

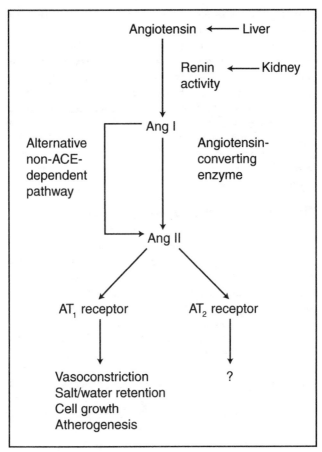

Figure 1: The renin-angiotensin system.

the importance of the AT_2 receptor in health and disease remains largely speculative.

Initial reports of the RAS describe a system based in the circulation. In this classical RAS system, angiotensinogen is released from the liver into the circulation, where it comes into contact with circulating renin activity that originates in the kidney. The resultant Ang I is acted on by ACE at the endothelial cell surface. The Ang II that is generated is then transported, within the bloodstream, throughout the body, where it comes into contact with the angiotensin receptors. In this way, the circulatory RAS system allows widespread distribution of Ang II throughout the body. There is little question that activation of this system contributes to the development and progression of cardiac dysfunction and to the hemodynamic abnormalities that characterize heart failure. However, there is now evidence that many of the effects of the RAS are also related to activation of a second tissue-based system.

Expression of the genes for ACE and angiotensin receptors occurs in the organs, such as the heart, kidney, and blood vessels.[5-9] Moreover, evidence shows that the level of expression is increased in settings that lead to or are associated with heart failure.[10] Although renin activity has also been detected in tissue, it is not clear whether this key proteolytic enzyme is generated locally or whether it is extracted from the circulating pool of renin activity by the tissue. An additional characteristic of the tissue-based RAS is that alternative pathways for the generation of Ang II from Ang I bypass the classical pathway that uses ACE (Figure 1). Perhaps the best characterized alternative pathway is the one that uses chymase, a proteolytic enzyme released from mast cells.[11-13] Although the relative importance of the tissue-based RAS compared to the circulatory systems is not yet fully defined, evidence shows that it may contribute substantially to the generation of Ang II in the heart and other organs.

Effects of Ang II

As outlined in Table 1, Ang II has a wide portfolio of effects relevant to the development and progression of heart failure. It is important to recognize that Ang II has not only short-term hemodynamic effects that can lead to and substantially worsen heart failure, but also long-

Table 1: Effects of Angiotensin II

- Vasoconstriction
- Salt/water retention (via aldosterone)
- Stimulation of vasopressin and norepinephrine release
- Renal efferent arteriolar vasoconstriction
- Cardiac myocyte hypertrophy
- Myocyte necrosis
- Fibroblast proliferation, migration, and collagen production
- Release of secondary growth factors (eg, TGF-β, ET)
- Production of free oxygen radicals
- Vascular smooth muscle proliferation and hypertrophy
- Decreased fibrinolysis (through increased vascular PAI-1 production)

TGF-β = transforming growth factor-β
ET = endothelin
PAI-1= plasminogen activator inhibitor-1

term effects that are involved in conditions such as hypertension, LVH, atherosclerosis, and coronary artery thrombosis, all of which result in cardiac dysfunction. An important aspect of these long-term effects of Ang II is the role that this growth-promoting peptide plays in the remodeling of the heart, leading to progressive cardiac dysfunction.

Hemodynamic Effects of Ang II

Initially, the most important aspects of Ang II were its effects on blood vessels, which promoted constriction of arterial resistance vessels, and its effects on renal hemodynamics and function, which resulted in salt and water retention. These effects are clearly important in the pathogenesis of heart failure, particularly in patients with advanced cardiac dysfunction. Most of these effects are immediate, and they are subject to rapid modulation by the concentration of Ang II. These hemodynamic effects are largely mediated by the classical circulatory RAS and tend to be compensatory changes that develop to augment cardiac output and/or increase perfusion pressure to vital organs. Additional immediate effects of the RAS that are relevant to the pathogenesis of heart failure include presynaptic stimulation of sympathetic nerves to enhance norepinephrine release and stimulation of thirst through release of arginine vasopressin.

Atherogenic/Profibrotic/Thrombogenic Effects

In blood vessels, Ang II causes endothelial cell dysfunction and vascular smooth muscle proliferation and growth. It also enhances fibroblast proliferation and activation that leads to deposition of extracellular matrix (ECM) within the vessel wall. Many of these latter effects appear to be mediated through Ang II stimulation of secondary growth factors, including transforming growth factor-β (TGF-β). The net effect of these properties of Ang II is to promote plaque growth and instability. Ang II also has antifibrinolytic properties related largely to its ability to stimulate the production of plasminogen activator inhibitor-1 (PAI-1).[14] As explained later in this chapter, interventions that block the RAS in patients with manifest atherosclerotic disease (or in those at high risk for this condition) have highly significant reductions in future events that lead to heart failure and increase patient survival.

Effects of Ang II on Remodeling

Evidence now shows that Ang II is a growth factor for cardiac myocytes and fibroblasts.[15-17] Consequently, Ang

II is believed to play a role in promoting the development of LVH, a condition resulting in systolic and diastolic heart dysfunction and, later, in frank heart failure. Patients who experience myocardial injury often undergo cardiac remodeling, which is most likely to occur if the amount of damage is significant or if increases in load on the heart persist over an extended period.[18,19] Remodeling can occur after myocardial infarction (MI), as a consequence of long-standing pressure or volume overload (as occurs in the setting of hypertension or long-standing valvular heart disease), or as a result of myocyte damage caused by such conditions as viral infection of the heart, alcohol abuse, or use of drugs such as doxorubicin (Adriamycin®). An important characteristic of the remodeling process is that it often continues well after the initial inciting event has resolved. Remodeling involves increases in LV volume and mass, as well as changes in conformation that ultimately lead to systolic and diastolic dysfunction. Additionally, there is substantial and convincing evidence that the RAS plays an important role in progressive remodeling in many of these settings.

Patterns of Activation of the RAS

In considering the role of the RAS in the pathogenesis of heart failure, system activation may be continuous throughout the life of the patient or it can be triggered by events that alter internal homeostasis. These 'triggers' of the RAS are often events that alter cardiac function and/or tissue perfusion pressure. The former, however, is related to a series of alternate gene forms or to polymorphisms in the genes that encode key proteins of the RAS (Table 2).[20-24] These polymorphisms give rise to proteins that have different functional capacities, which, in some cases, result in enhanced RAS activity or effects. Perhaps the best studied of these polymorphisms is the one for the ACE gene, in which the DD allele confers a higher degree of enzyme activity and, by inference, increased generation of Ang II. The presence of this allele was first associated with increased risk of MI,[20] presumably based on the effects of Ang II in promoting atherogenesis and thrombosis. The DD phenotype has now also been associated with increased incidence of hypertension, LVH, and heart failure,[23-25] as well as with increased mortality in patients with cardiac disease.[26]

More commonly, however, activation of the RAS develops when the internal milieu of the patient is upset and cardiac output and/or arterial perfusion pressure are reduced. When this occurs, activation of the RAS helps reset the equilibrium mainly by promoting peripheral arterial vasoconstriction and salt and water retention. As a primitive mechanism to temporarily preserve perfusion of vital organs, this is highly effective and has great compensatory benefits in situations where the life of the patient is threatened by either dehydration or blood loss. For the reasons outlined in Table 1, however, the long-term activation of the RAS in the setting of cardiac dysfunction is highly undesirable because it ultimately promotes further worsening in cardiac performance and is a major factor in the deleterious remodeling that leads to progressive cardiac dysfunction.

Activation patterns of classical or circulatory RAS in the natural history of heart failure have now been reasonably well delineated.[27-32] Following an abrupt change in cardiac function, such as the one occurring after MI, there is an initial activation of the RAS, as evidenced by an increase in plasma renin activity. With resolution of the acute event, however, this system becomes quiescent again unless there is a reduction in cardiac output and/or blood pressure. Patients with asymptomatic LV dysfunction have little evidence of circulatory RAS activation unless they are receiving diuretic agents that are known to stimulate release of plasma renin activity from the kidney.[30] As heart failure develops, plasma renin activity goes up, and, generally, the severity of heart failure symptoms is roughly paralleled by the extent of the rise in plasma renin activity, so that patients with the greatest evidence of decompensation have the highest levels of plasma renin activity.[27,31]

LV dysfunction tends to be progressive, mainly as a consequence of ongoing cardiac remodeling. The description of changes in plasma renin activity might give the impression that RAS involvement in the development of heart failure does not happen until evidence of decompensation occurs. Evidence derived mainly from experimental animal models that demonstrates early and continuous activation of the tissue-based cardiac RAS indicates that this is not the case. Much of this information comes from various animal models of MI. In this setting, increased ACE activity and augmented levels of Ang II have been demonstrated within the myocardium, even when plasma renin activity is not elevated.[28,29,32-34] Additionally, evidence shows that the density of the AT_1 receptor is increased in the post-MI setting;[35-37] interestingly, this up-regulation of the AT_1 receptor appears to occur predominantly on cardiac fibroblasts.[38]

There is now evidence that this increase in AT_1 receptor density increases fibroblast functions that favor the deposition of ECM.[39] Thus, cardiac RAS activation plays a major role in the progressive remodeling of the heart that takes place after injury and leads to worsening cardiac function.

Effects of Drug Therapies That Interrupt the RAS

ACE Inhibitors

The first available agents to block the RAS were the ACE inhibitors, which were initially developed to treat hypertension. Their efficacy in reducing blood pressure and the risk of end-organ damage is now well established. However, the beneficial effects of ACE inhibitors in treating patients with heart failure at virtually all levels of severity, post-MI patients, and patients at increased risk of developing heart failure because of the presence of atherosclerotic disease have now been recognized. Interestingly, as indications for the use of ACE inhibitors have grown, uncertainty about the mechanism(s) responsible for their ability to alter the natural history of important cardiovascular diseases has emerged. Much of the debate centers around the issue of the relative importance of the effects of ACE inhibitors in blocking the production of Ang II vs their effects in enhancing the levels of bradykinin.[40,41] At present, although no definitive answer to this question has emerged, data appear to show that both of these properties of ACE inhibitors may contribute to their beneficial effects.

ACE inhibitors in the prevention of cardiovascular events and heart failure. There is considerable evidence that the RAS plays an important role in the progression of atherosclerotic disease and in the likelihood of future cardiovascular events. The sources of this hypothesis include epidemiologic surveys indicating that hypertensive patients with high levels of plasma renin activity are at increased risk of cardiovascular events (ie, MI) and genetic studies

Table 3: Entry Criteria in the HOPE Study

- Men or women at 55 years of age
- History of coronary artery disease, stroke, peripheral vascular disease, or diabetes plus one other cardiovascular risk factor*
- Patients were excluded if they:
  - had heart failure
  - had an EF <0.40
  - were taking an ACE inhibitor or vitamin E
  - had uncontrolled hypertension or overt nephropathy
  - had an MI or stroke within 4 weeks

* Hypertension, elevated total cholesterol, low HDL cholesterol levels, cigarette smoking, or documented microalbuminuria.

HOPE = Heart Outcomes Prevention Evaluation

EF = ejection fraction

ACE = angiotensin-converting enzyme

MI = myocardial infarction

demonstrating that patients with the DD allele of the ACE gene are also at higher risk of MI.[20,42,43] Furthermore, post-hoc analysis of the results of the Studies of Left Ventricular Dysfunction (SOLVD) and Survival and Ventricular Enlargement (SAVE) studies suggests that patients randomized to ACE inhibitors experienced a highly significant reduction in the risk of MI and unstable angina.[44,45]

Definitive proof of the value of blocking the RAS in preventing cardiovascular events is now available from the results of the Heart Outcomes Prevention Evaluation (HOPE) study.[46] Entry criteria for HOPE are summarized in Table 3. This trial enrolled 9,297 patients older than 55 years of age who did not show manifest LV dysfunction. Patients were selected for inclusion if they were at an increased risk for future events based on presence of coronary, peripheral, or cerebrovascular disease or presence of diabetes and at least one other standard cardiovascular risk factor or evidence of microalbuminuria. Patients enrolled in the HOPE study were randomly assigned to receive either the ACE inhibitor ramipril (Altace®) 10 mg/d or placebo in addition to their other medications. The primary end point of the study was a composite of acute MI, stroke, and cardiovascular mortality.

HOPE participants were followed for 5 years—at the end of the study, the primary composite end point of MI, stroke, and death from cardiovascular causes was reduced by 22% ($P < 0.001$) in the patients randomized to ramipril (Figure 2). Each of the components of the composite end point was significantly affected by ACE inhibitor therapy. There was a reduction in acute MI of 20%, in stroke of 32%, and in cardiovascular death of 26% (all $P < 0.001$). Additionally, multiple secondary cardiovascular and other end points were predesignated in HOPE. These end points and the risk reduction (RR) achieved with ACE inhibition are summarized in Table 4. Overall, there was a striking reduction in most cardiovascular events, and, not surprisingly, the likelihood of developing heart failure was reduced by 23% ($P < 0.001$) with ramipril.

Although the results of the HOPE study were unequivocally in favor of ACE inhibitor therapy, the study did not provide information about the mechanism through which the significant reduction in cardiovascular events was achieved. Although blood pressure was reduced with ramipril, the magnitude of the change in this variable with the drug (3/2 mm Hg for systolic/diastolic pressures) does not seem to be a sufficient explanation for the magnitude of the reduction in cardiovascular events. Possible mechanisms involved in the effects of ramipril in the HOPE study are listed in Table 5. Despite the absence of information

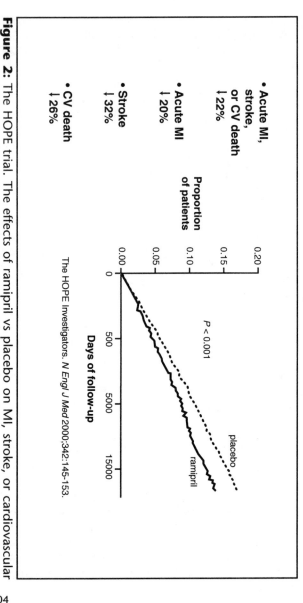

Figure 2: The HOPE trial. The effects of ramipril vs placebo on MI, stroke, or cardiovascular death in 9,297 high-risk patients without left ventricular dysfunction.

- **Acute MI, stroke, or CV death**
  ↓ 22%

- **Acute MI**
  ↓ 20%

- **Stroke**
  ↓ 32%

- **CV death**
  ↓ 26%

Proportion of patients

0.20
0.15
0.10
0.05
0.00

0   500   5000   15000

Days of follow-up

P < 0.001

placebo

ramipril

The HOPE Investigators. *N Engl J Med* 2000;342:145-153.

Table 4: Effects of Ramipril on Secondary and Other End Points of the HOPE Study

Secondary End Points	Risk Reduction (%)	*P* Value
Revascularization	15	0.002
Unstable angina hospitalization	2	NS
Diabetes complications	16	0.03
Heart failure hospitalizations	12	0.25

Other Outcomes	Risk Reduction (%)	*P* Value
Heart failure	23	<0.001
Cardiac arrest	38	0.02
Worsening angina	11	0.004
New diagnosis of diabetes	34	<0.001
Unstable angina with EKG changes	3	NS

NS = not studied
EKG = electrocardiogram

defining the mechanism of the protective effects of ACE inhibition with ramipril in these high-risk patients, there is no question about the implications of the HOPE study. The patients included in the trial are similar to those seen in most office and clinic practices, and the results provide persuasive evidence that such high-risk patients will ben-

Table 5: Potential Mechanism(s) Responsible for the Reduction of Events in HOPE

- Blood pressure reduction
- Reduced vasoconstriction
- Decreased proliferation of vascular smooth muscle cells
- Increased plaque stability
- Improved vascular endothelium function
- Reduced left ventricular hypertrophy
- Enhanced fibrinolysis

efit substantially from ACE inhibitor therapy. Thus, in patients who fulfill HOPE entry criteria, an ACE inhibitor is strongly advised unless there is a contraindication to such therapy. If this suggestion was implemented throughout the high-risk population, approximately 150 events in 70 patients would be prevented for every 1,000 patients treated over a 4-year period.

ACE inhibitors post-MI. Several studies have been designed to assess the efficacy of ACE inhibitors post-MI.[45,47-51] These studies mostly enrolled patients who had evidence of substantial LV damage, although some patients were asymptomatic while others had evidence of heart failure at the time of randomization to an ACE inhibitor or placebo. Despite differences in entry criteria and in the drug used, the studies showed remarkable consistency in their results. All of these trials demonstrated significant reductions in all-cause mortality with ACE inhibitor therapy compared to standard therapy. Overall, the reduction in mortality was 20% to 25% with ACE inhibitor therapy.

In SAVE, patients with an ejection fraction (EF) <0.40 after MI were randomized to captopril (eg, Capoten®,

Acenorm®) 50 mg t.i.d. or placebo in addition to their other medications.[45] Captopril therapy was associated with a 19% reduction in all-cause mortality (P=0.019), the primary end point of the study. Cardiovascular mortality was reduced by 21%, and recurrent MI was reduced by 25%. The development of heart failure was designated as a secondary end point of the SAVE study, and overall, there was a significant 37% RR (P=0.032) associated with captopril treatment (Figure 3). Another example is the Acute Infarction Ramipril Efficiency (AIRE) study.[52] In this trial, patients with clinical evidence of heart failure post-MI were randomized to either ramipril or placebo. The results of the AIRE study showed that ACE inhibitor therapy reduced all-cause mortality by 27% (P=0.002) and the combined end point of death, severe or resistant congestive heart failure (CHF), reinfarction, and stroke by 19% (P=0.008).

ACE inhibitors in patients with asymptomatic LV dysfunction. The prevention arm of SOLVD studied the effects of ACE inhibition in patients with asymptomatic LV dysfunction (ie, LVEF <0.35).[53] Although most patients (more than 80% in the enalapril [Vasotec®] and placebo groups) had underlying coronary artery disease as the cause of their LV dysfunction, entry into the study was precluded for at least 6 months post-MI. Thus, the SOLVD prevention arm population was distinctly different from the patients included in studies evaluating ACE inhibition in the immediate post-MI period. Additionally, a substantial number of patients with a nonischemic etiology of their heart failure were included in the study. The 4,228 patients included in the prevention arm of SOLVD were assigned to receive either enalapril 10 mg b.i.d. or placebo in addition to their other medications. Although there was an 8% reduction in the primary end point of all-cause mortality, the results did not achieve statistical significance. However, after an average of 3 years' follow-up, death or hospitalization because of heart failure was re-

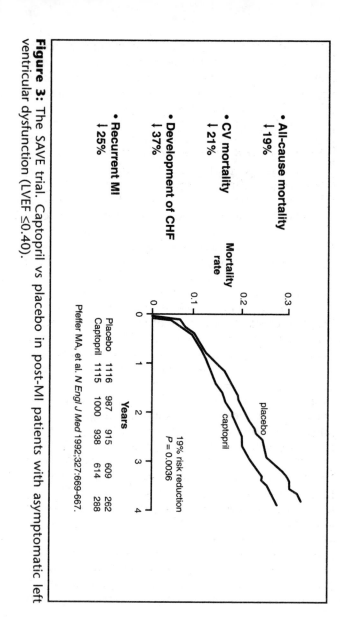

Figure 3: The SAVE trial. Captopril vs placebo in post-MI patients with asymptomatic left ventricular dysfunction (LVEF ≤0.40).

• All-cause mortality
↓ 19%

• CV mortality
↓ 21%

• Development of CHF
↓ 37%

• Recurrent MI
↓ 25%

19% risk reduction
P = 0.0036

placebo

captopril

Mortality rate

Years

	0	1	2	3	4
Placebo	1116	987	915	609	262
Captopril	1115	1000	938	614	288

Pfeffer MA, et al. *N Engl J Med* 1992;327:669-667.

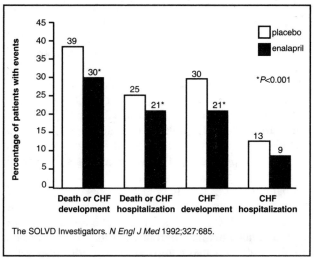

Figure 4: SOLVD prevention trial. Enalapril vs placebo in 4,228 patients with asymptomatic left ventricular dysfunction (LVEF ≤35%).

duced by 20%, death or development of heart failure was reduced by 29%, development of heart failure was reduced by 37%, and heart failure hospitalizations were reduced by 44% (all *P*<0.001), as shown in Figure 4.

ACE inhibitors in patients with symptomatic LV dysfunction. The treatment arm of SOLVD assessed the effects of ACE inhibitors in patients with mild to moderate symptoms of heart failure associated with a reduced LVEF.[54] The study included 2,579 patients with heart failure from either ischemic or nonischemic causes. As in the prevention arm, patients were randomly assigned to receive either enalapril 10 mg b.i.d. or placebo in addition to their other heart failure medications, such as digoxin (Lanoxin®), diuretics (eg, furosemide [Lasix®]), and non-ACE inhibitor vasodilators. After an average 3.5-year follow-up, there was a highly significant 16% reduction (*P*=0.0036) in all-cause mortality, the primary end point of the study (Figure 5). Cardiovascular hospitalizations were reduced by 10%, death caused by progressive heart failure was reduced by 22%, and death or heart failure hospitalizations were reduced by 26% ($P<0.00001$).

Effects of ACE inhibitors on LV remodeling in the SOLVD study. As part of SOLVD, a group of 300 representative patients underwent serial echo-Doppler evaluation over the course of the first 12 months after randomization to ACE inhibitor or placebo.[55] The study included prevention- and treatment-arm patients, and the results were pooled together when analysis showed no significant interaction between the effects of therapy and the patient arm of the study. The results of the changes in cardiac structure with ACE inhibitor therapy are summarized in Table 6. They show that at baseline, LV volumes and mass in this subgroup of SOLVD patients were considerably elevated compared with a control population, indicating that the study patients had already undergone substantial amounts of LV remodeling. Over the 12-month follow-up period, significant increases in LV volume and mass occurred in the patients randomized to placebo. These results show that cardiac remodeling in patients with LV dysfunction is a progressive process and that the adverse changes in cardiac structure continue to develop over an extended period. Patients treated with enalapril, however, demonstrated inhibition of further increase in LV volume or mass. Over the course of the study, the differences in the changes in LV structure between the placebo- and enalapril-treated patients were significant. These results show the protective effect of ACE inhibition on progressive LV remodeling. They suggest that the beneficial effects of enalapril on the natural history of patients with LV dysfunction seen in the SOLVD trials are partly the result of enalapril's ability to prevent further heart remodeling from occurring.

ACE inhibitors in patients with advanced LV dysfunction. Patients enrolled in the Cooperative North Scandina-

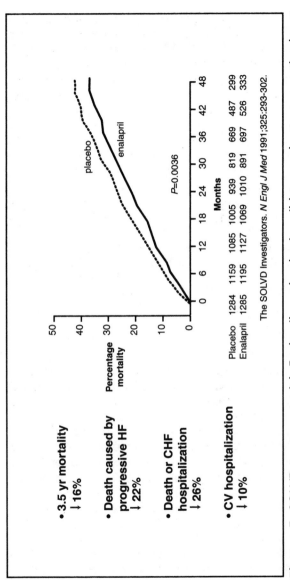

Figure 5: SOLVD treatment trial. Enalapril vs placebo in mild to moderate congestive heart failure (CHF) with LVEF ≤0.35.

- **3.5 yr mortality** ↓ 16%
- **Death caused by progressive HF** ↓ 22%
- **Death or CHF hospitalization** ↓ 26%
- **CV hospitalization** ↓ 10%

P=0.0036

placebo

enalapril

Percentage mortality

Months

	0	6	12	18	24	30	36	42	48
Placebo	1284	1159	1085	1005	939	819	669	487	299
Enalapril	1285	1195	1127	1069	1010	891	697	526	333

The SOLVD Investigators. *N Engl J Med* 1991;325:293-302.

Table 6: Effects of Enalapril on Cardiac Remodeling in SOLVD

Variable	Treatment	Baseline
EDV (mL)	P	200 ± 42
	E	196 ± 41
	C	131 ± 30
ESV (mL)	P	148 ± 38
	E	146 ± 38
	C	64 ± 25
LV mass (g)	P	280 ± 100
	E	265 ± 82
	C	133 ± 45

EDV = end-diastolic volume; ESV = end-systolic volume; LV = left ventricular; P = placebo; E = enalapril; C = control; B = baseline.

vian Enalapril Survival Study (CONSENSUS) had New York Heart Association (NYHA) Class IV symptoms of heart failure together with LV systolic dysfunction. The 253 patients enrolled in this trial were randomly assigned to receive either enalapril or placebo in addition to their standard heart failure therapy. Confirmation of heart failure severity in the CONSENSUS population came from the observation that mortality in the placebo-treated patients was approximately 50% at 6 months.[56] The addition of an ACE inhibitor had a profound influence on the clinical course of these patients. Enalapril reduced 6-month mortality by 40% ($P=0.002$) and 1-year mortality by 31% ($P=0.001$). Death caused by progressive heart failure was reduced by 50% ($P=0.001$). Additionally, evidence showed

P value 12 Months	P value (B vs 12M)	(P vs E)
210 ± 46	0.003	0.025
197 ± 39	0.852	
156 ± 42	0.014	0.019
145 ± 38	0.594	
297 ± 100	0.178	<0.001
255 ± 82	0.280	

that enalapril reduced NYHA class, heart size, and medication use in the CONSENSUS study population.

Recommendations for the use of ACE inhibitors in the prevention and treatment of heart failure. All of the trials described were double-blinded, placebo-controlled, and adequately sized to assess morbidity and mortality end points. Based on these results, recommendations regarding the use of ACE inhibitors can be offered (Table 7). Basically, ACE inhibitors should be used in a broad spectrum of patients who either have heart failure or are at risk for developing it. Their value is more extensive than was initially thought when the drugs were first approved to treat patients with symptomatic heart failure. Now there is compelling evidence that ACE inhibitor use should ex-

Table 7: Recommendations for the Use of ACE Inhibitors to Prevent and/or Treat Heart Failure

- Post-MI patients regardless of EF
- Patients with diabetes and one of the following:
  - hypertension
  - elevated total cholesterol
  - low HDL cholesterol
  - cigarette smoking
  - presence of microalbuminuria
- NYHA Class II, III, IV heart failure
- Asymptomatic LV dysfunction with an EF ≤ 0.40

ACE = angiotensin-converting enzyme
EF = ejection fraction
MI = myocardial infarction
HDL = high-density lipoprotein
NYHA = New York Heart Association
LV = left ventricular

tend all the way from patients who are at risk for cardio-vascular events to those who have severe NYHA Class IV symptoms of heart failure. This includes MI survivors and patients with LV dysfunction regardless of symptomatic state.

An overview of the initiation and maintenance of ACE inhibitors is shown in Table 8. These drugs are usually initiated at a low dose and then up-titrated to the desired dose over a few days to weeks. The initial and optimal doses of approved ACE inhibitors are shown in Table 9. Before initiation of therapy, patients should have blood drawn for measurement of electrolytes and renal function. Patients with hyperkalemia should not begin taking the ACE inhibitor until this condition has been satisfactorily treated

Table 8: Initiation and Maintenance of ACE Inhibitors

- Assess patient's volume status, serum electrolytes, and renal function before initiation of therapy.

- Do not start therapy in patients with symptomatic hypotension, hyperkalemia, or severe renal failure.

- Initiate ACE inhibitors at a low dose and gradually up-titrate to optimal dose.

- Repeat measurement of electrolytes and renal function after initiation of therapy and after optimal dosing regimen has been achieved.

and it is clear that the cause of the high potassium levels has been corrected. Abnormal renal function is a relative contraindication to the use of ACE inhibitors since the effects of these drugs on blood pressure and intrarenal hemodynamics are likely to result in a worsening of this condition. However, most heart failure experts will initiate therapy with ACE inhibitors in patients with serum creatinine levels <2.5 to 3.0 mg/dL. Although a further rise in the creatinine level is likely to occur, it is important to recognize that this does not indicate irreversible renal damage, but rather altered kidney function that can usually be reversed with discontinuation of the ACE inhibitor. This chemical abnormality needs to be considered in the context of the long-term clinical benefits of ACE inhibitor therapy. In most cases, the risk/benefit ratio falls on the side of using the drugs unless there is a >30% increase in serum creatinine levels or the level is elevated above 3.0 mg/dL. In these cases, it may be advisable to reduce or discontinue the ACE inhibitor or to adjust the diuretic dose.

Many heart failure patients have abnormally low blood pressure when initiation of ACE inhibitors is being considered. This has been a common and, in most cases, unneces-

Table 9: ACE Inhibitors Approved for Treatment of Heart Failure and LV Dysfunction

Agent	HF	LV Dysfunction	Dose
captopril (Capoten®)	√	√ (post-MI)	6.25 mg- 50 mg t.i.d.
enalapril (Vasotec®)	√	√ (asymptomatic)	2.5 mg- 10 mg b.i.d.
fosinopril (Monopril®)	√	NA	20 mg- 40 mg q.d.
lisinopril (Prinivil®, Zestril®)	√	NA	5 mg- 20 mg q.d.
quinapril (Accupril®)	√	NA	10 mg- 20 mg b.i.d.
ramipril (Altace®)	√	√ (post-MI)	5 mg b.i.d.
trandolapril (Mavik®)	√	√ (post-MI)	1 mg- 4 mg q.d.

Indication spans HF and LV Dysfunction columns.

ACE = angiotensin-converting enzyme
LV = left ventricular
HF = heart failure
MI = myocardial infarction

sary impediment to the implementation of this highly beneficial therapy. The absolute level of blood pressure should not be used to determine if a patient can be started on an ACE inhibitor, nor should it be used to determine the optimal dose of the drug for that patient. A more rational method is to determine if the blood pressure at the time of therapy initiation (and after each successive dose) is tolerated by the patient. The decision to stop an ACE inhibitor, maintain the drug at a less-than-optimal dose, or reduce the dose should be based on whether there is evidence of tissue hypoperfusion. This is usually manifested by either lightheadedness and dizziness (caused by cerebral hypoperfusion) or by more serious evidence of renal dysfunction than outlined earlier. This approach allows appropriate up-titration of the drug in patients who appear to have borderline blood pressures and provides guidelines for restraint in dosing patients who cannot tolerate therapy despite 'normal' blood pressure.

Angioedema is a serious side effect of ACE inhibitor therapy that can be life-threatening in severe cases. Its prevalence is estimated to be <1%, but it is more common in African Americans. Angioedema appears to be mediated by increased bradykinin, particularly in genetically predisposed persons. The appearance of angioedema is an indication to permanently discontinue ACE inhibitor therapy. Cough is a troublesome side effect of the ACE inhibitors that occurs in approximately 5% to 10% of patients. However, its incidence may be higher in selected populations. It is important to distinguish ACE inhibitor-mediated cough from cough caused by other reasons in the heart failure population. Continuation of cough after other causes have been excluded may be a reason to discontinue therapy in some patients with severe symptoms.

Angiotensin-Receptor Blockers in the Treatment of Heart Failure

Angiotensin-receptor blockers (ARBs) are a relatively new class of drugs used to block the RAS. They are pharmacologically distinct from ACE inhibitors and offer an alternative means for blocking the effects of Ang II.[57,58] ARBs, in contrast to ACE inhibitors, block the interaction between Ang II and the AT_1 receptor regardless of the source of the peptide. Thus, it is irrelevant whether Ang II was generated by ACE or through an alternative pathway that uses enzymes such as chymase. However, ACE inhibitors have additional effects that are potentially important in the pathogenesis of cardiovascular disease; they also block the breakdown of bradykinin, a peptide with effects that may be relevant to the pathogenesis of a variety of cardiovascular diseases.[59,60] For example, bradykinin causes relaxation of vascular smooth muscle by stimulating the release of prostacyclin and nitric oxide (NO) from endothelial cells lining the luminal surface of blood vessels. Bradykinin is also believed to have antigrowth effects on cardiac cells. Consequently, it may inhibit cardiac and vascular hypertrophy and remodeling. Thus, in some ways, bradykinin acts directionally opposite to Ang II. However, other properties of bradykinin may not be so favorable. Bradykinin is believed to be the agent responsible for ACE-inhibitor induced cough, a troublesome side effect of this class of drugs. It also stimulates release of norepinephrine. In the heart failure setting, where elevated levels of catecholamines are known to be important in the progression of disease, this a highly undesirable property.

ARB therapy to prevent heart failure. The use of ARB therapy to prevent progression of disease and as a way to reduce risk has been assessed in patients with type II diabetes, proteinuria, and elevated serum creatinine levels in the Reduction of End Points in Non-Insulin Dependent Diabetes Mellitus with the Angiotensin II Antagonist Losartan (RENAAL) trial. Of the 1,513 patients enrolled in RENAAL, 92% had hypertension in addition to diabetes. Although these patients were receiving a variety of drugs to treat their hypertension, the use of an ACE inhibitor or an ARB at the time of randomization was not allowed. Patients who met the entry criteria were randomized to receive placebo or losartan (Hyzaar®, Cozaar®) 50 to 100 mg q.d. in addition to their other medications. Over a mean follow-up period of 3.4 years, fewer patients discontinued losartan than placebo (17% vs 22%). The primary end point of this study was a composite of end-stage renal disease (ESRD), a two-fold increase in serum creatinine level, or death. The results of RENAAL are sum-

Table 10: Results of RENAAL

- Primary composite end point (eg, doubling of serum creatinine; ESRD; death) was reduced 16% (P=0.024) with losartan

- Losartan reduced the components of the primary end point as follows:
  - 28% reduction in ESRD (P=0.002)
  - 25% reduction in doubling serum creatinine (P=0.006)
  - no significant mortality effect
  - 20% reduction in death or ESRD (P=0.010)

- Addition of losartan affected other end points:
  - 35% reduction in proteinuria (P=0.000)
  - 32% reduction in HF hospitalization (P=0.005)

RENAAL = Reduction of End Points in Non-Insulin-Dependent Diabetes Mellitus with the Angiotensin II Antagonist Losartan
ESRD = end-stage renal disease
HF = heart failure

marized in Table 10. At the time that the study was stopped, there was a 16% reduction in the primary composite end point in the losartan-treated patients.

This effect of losartan was statistically significant and was caused predominantly by the protective effects of losartan on renal function, as evidenced by the 28% reduction in ESRD and the 25% reduction in the likelihood of increased creatinine levels. Thus, the addition of losartan to this high-risk, mostly diabetic, hypertensive population reduced the future likelihood of deterioration in renal function. Based on the presence of potent cardiovascular risk factors, clinicians would anticipate that the RENAAL population would be at relatively high risk for developing heart failure. The addition of losartan, however, reduced this risk considerably, as evidenced by the 32% reduction in heart failure hospitalizations (P=0.005) compared to the placebo group.

ARBs as alternatives to ACE inhibitors in the treatment of heart failure. The possibility that treatment with an ARB might have more favorable effects on survival in heart failure patients was assessed in the Evaluation of Losartan in the Elderly II (ELITE II) study.[61] There was great enthusiasm for this possibility based on the results of the ELITE I study, a trial that had unexpectedly demonstrated a nearly 50% lower mortality with losartan compared to captopril in elderly ACE inhibitor-naive patients.[62] Interestingly, ELITE I had not been designed to assess mortality as an end point of the study. The primary end point of ELITE I was the effect of an ARB vs an ACE inhibitor on renal function in a heart failure population. The results of ELITE I demonstrated conclusively that there was essentially no significant difference in the likelihood of a clinically important rise in serum creatinine between the treatments. Thus, the ELITE I study demonstrated that both ACEs and ARBs were well tolerated by the kidneys. The ELITE II study was then constructed to test the hypothesis that losartan 50 mg q.d. would reduce mortality by 20% when compared to a control population that was treated with the ACE inhibitor captopril 50 mg t.i.d. Patients enrolled in ELITE II were older than 54 years of age and were ACE inhibitor naive. They were required to have symptomatic heart failure (ie, NYHA Class II-IV) and an LVEF <0.40. The results of the study did not support the hypothesis that losartan had a more favorable effect on mortality than captopril. As shown in Figure 6, the life table curves for the two treatment regimens for all-cause mortality, the primary end point of the study, were not significantly different. For secondary end points, such as quality of life and NYHA class, there were significant improvements with either drug and no significant differences in the response between them. The changes in quality of life from baseline with the two

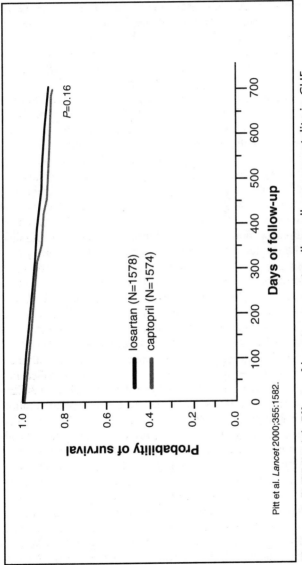

Figure 6: ELITE II trial. Effects of losartan vs captopril on all-cause mortality in CHF.

Pitt et al. *Lancet* 2000;355:1582.

therapies are summarized in Figure 7. Losartan, however, was better tolerated than captopril. Withdrawals and the reasons for drug discontinuation because of adverse advents with losartan and captopril are shown in Figure 8.

Effects of combined ACE inhibitor and ARB therapy. The Valsartan in Heart Failure Trial (Val-HeFT) study was designed to determine if the combination of an ARB and an ACE inhibitor significantly improved the natural history of patients with heart failure compared to the effects of ACE inhibitor therapy alone. Val-HeFT included patients with evidence of LV dysfunction and symptomatic heart failure despite standard therapy, including an ACE inhibitor. Patients were randomly assigned to either placebo or to valsartan (Diovan®) started at 40 mg b.i.d. and titrated to 160 mg b.i.d. The two primary end points of the trial were all-cause mortality and combined mortality and morbidity. The results of the study are summarized in Table 11. No significant benefit in mortality reduction was seen with combined therapy compared to ACE inhibitor treatment alone. However, the combined mortality and morbidity end point was reduced by 13.3% ($P=0.009$) by the addition of valsartan to the ACE inhibitor. As shown in Figure 9, this reduction was largely caused by a highly significant 27.5% reduction in heart failure hospitalization with combined ARB/ACE inhibitor therapy.

Subgroup analysis of the results of Val-HeFT has provided important insights into the clinical application of ARBs in the treatment of patients with heart failure. These results are summarized in Figure 10. In the 7% of the Val-HeFT patients who were not taking ACE inhibitors, the administration of valsartan had a substantial impact in reducing combined mortality and morbidity by 44% ($P<0.0002$). These results provide much-needed information about the effects of ARB therapy in heart failure, since there is a paucity of placebo-controlled data assessing the effects of ARBs alone. The predefined subgroup analysis also looked at the interaction of ARB and ACE inhibitor

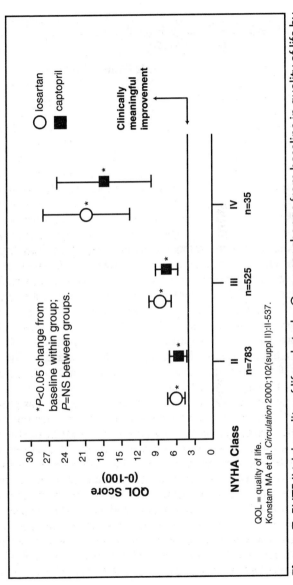

Figure 7: ELITE II trial quality of life substudy. One-year change from baseline in quality of life by NYHA class among survivors.

QOL = quality of life.
Konstam MA et al. *Circulation* 2000;102(suppl II):II-537.

Table 11: Primary End Points in Val-HeFT

Event	Valsartan (N=2,511)	Placebo (N=2,499)
All-cause mortality	495 (19.7%)	484 (19.4%)
Combined all-cause mortality and morbidity	723 (28.8%)	801 (32.1%)

therapy with β-blocker therapy. Unfortunately, only 35% of the Val-HeFT patients were receiving a β-blocker. There was, however, evidence of an interaction, since patients not receiving the β-blocker who were randomized to valsartan did significantly better than those who were receiving a β-blocker. In the latter group, there was a trend toward an unfavorable outcome when patients were receiving all three agents. However, the confidence intervals extended over the neutrality line, so this interaction was not statistically significant. Overall, the subgroup results suggest that the addition of an ARB is more likely to be effective in patients who are not receiving optimal neurohormonal blockade with other agents. The data also discourage the concept of adding an ARB to the regimen of a patient who is already on a combination of ACE inhibitor and β-blocker therapy.

Other clinical trials with ARBs in heart failure. The Randomized Evaluation of Strategies for Left Ventricular Dysfunction (RESOLVD) pilot study was designed to provide information about the effects of candesartan (Atacand®) compared to enalapril and added to an ACE inhibitor on a variety of heart failure end points.[63] The study included multiple doses of both drugs. During the course of the trial, further randomization to the β-blocker metoprolol (Toprol-XL®) or to placebo was carried out. Combined treatment with candesartan and an ACE inhibitor resulted in a greater increase in LVEF and less of an

RR (CI)	P value
1.02 (0.90-1.15)	0.800
0.87 (0.79-0.96)	0.009

increase in LV systolic and diastolic volumes than with either drug alone. The results showed no significant difference in mortality, hospitalizations for CHF, or hospitalizations for any cause among the three groups. However, the study was not adequately powered for determining differences in these events between the various therapeutic regimens. The overall results of the RESOLVD pilot study are consistent with the possibility that combined ACE inhibitor and ARB therapy might be a better way to inhibit LV remodeling than therapy with either drug alone.

Role of ARBs in preventing and treating heart failure. Recommendations for the use of ARBs in treating patients with heart failure are outlined in Table 12. It is important to recognize that our ability to obtain definitive information about the role of ARBs in the treatment of heart failure has been hampered by the fact that ARBs were developed after ACE inhibitors had already been established as a standard of heart failure therapy. With the large number of clinical trials (some of which are described previously) demonstrating the efficacy of ACE inhibitors and their overall acceptance into the therapeutic regimen, studies comparing an ARB to placebo have been difficult to perform. Since many trials have demonstrated the substantial clinical efficacy of ACE inhibitors in the treatment of patients with heart failure, there is no compelling

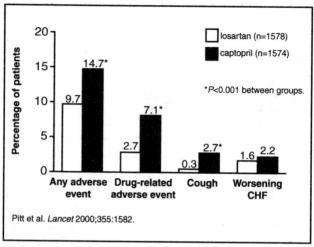

Figure 8: ELITE II trial. Withdrawals because of adverse effects.

reason to substitute an ARB for an ACE inhibitor if a patient tolerates the latter class of drugs. However, the results from ELITE I and II that show no significant difference between an ACE inhibitor and an ARB for either a renal end point or in mortality support the conclusion that ACE inhibitor-intolerant patients should receive an ARB as second-line therapy for the treatment of heart failure. The important but limited information (because of the small size of the subgroup) from the Val-HeFT patients who were not receiving an ACE inhibitor show an improved clinical course with valsartan and support this recommendation.

The use of combined ACE inhibitor and ARB therapy in heart failure remains somewhat controversial. The Val-HeFT study results demonstrate significant improvement in the combined primary mortality/morbidity end point, as evidenced by a significant reduction in heart failure hospitalizations. A 27% reduction in heart failure hospitalization rate is highly desirable, since hospitalization costs con-

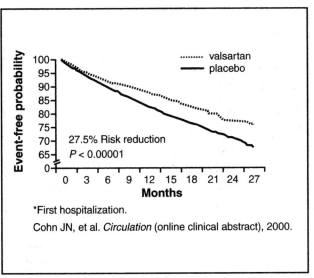

Figure 9: Val-HeFT. Heart failure hospitalizations.

sume roughly 60% to 70% of the money spent on heart failure in the United States. Whether there is an unfavorable interaction between ACE inhibitors, ARBs, and β-blockers in heart failure patients, as suggested in the Val-HeFT subgroup analysis, is uncertain at this time. However, since the Val-HeFT results provide no evidence of benefit from the addition of an ARB to patients already receiving an ACE inhibitor and a β-blocker, there is no compelling reason at this time to advocate this approach. Further information about the effects of adding an ARB to patients already on an ACE inhibitor and a β-blocker is clearly needed to help resolve this issue.

Future directions with ARBs in heart failure. As outlined in Table 12, the indications for the use of ARBs in the treatment of heart failure are still emerging. Clearly, more information is needed to better understand where and how to use this class of agents. The Candesartan

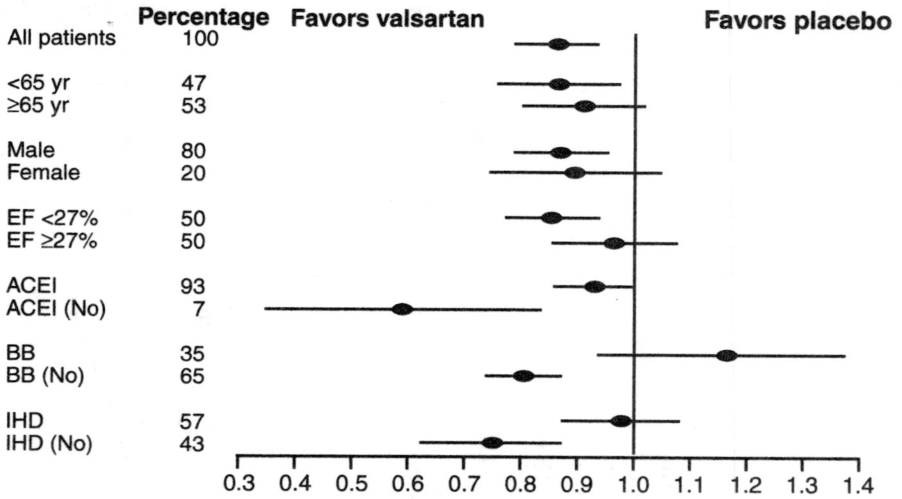
Percentage
Favors valsartan
Favors placebo
All patients 100
<65 yr 47
≥65 yr 53
Male 80
Female 20
EF <27% 50
EF ≥27% 50
ACEI 93
ACEI (No) 7
BB 35
BB (No) 65
IHD 57
IHD (No) 43
0.3 0.4 0.5 0.6 0.7 0.8 0.9 1.0 1.1 1.2 1.3 1.4

BB=β–blocker; IHD=ischemic heart disease; ACEI = ACE inhibitor.
Cohn: AHA 73rd Scientific Sessions, Nov 2000.

Figure 10: Val-HeFT. Combined morbidity/mortality in subgroups.

Table 12: Uses of ARBs in Treating Heart Failure

- As a substitute for an ACE inhibitor in patients with heart failure who cannot tolerate an ACE inhibitor

- As an addition to ACE inhibitors in patients who cannot tolerate a β-blocker

- As an alternative to an ACE inhibitor in patients with type 2 diabetes to prevent progression of renal disease and/or heart failure

- Treatment of patients with heart failure and preserved systolic function (speculative—this hypothesis is being tested in the CHARM study)

ARB = angiotensin-receptor blocker
ACE = angiotensin-converting enzyme
CHARM = Candesartan Cilexetil in Heart Failure Assessment of Reduction in Mortality and Morbidity

Cilexetil in Heart Failure Assessment of Reduction in Mortality and Morbidity (CHARM) study is a series of related but independent clinical trials assessing the effects of the ARB candesartan (Atacand®) in patients with heart failure. The three arms of the CHARM program are outlined in Table 13. The study arm in ACE-intolerant patients will provide extremely important and unique information that evaluates the effects of an ARB on the clinical course of patients with systolic dysfunction. At present, only limited placebo-controlled data addressing this question (eg, the results from the small subsegment of the Val-HeFT population that was not on an ACE inhibitor) are available. The arm assessing the effects of candesartan in addition to an ACE inhibitor will help provide better definition about the use of combined ACE inhibitor/ARB therapy in this population. Since a large segment of the

Table 13: The CHARM Study

Patient Populations	N value
LVEF ≤0.40	2,300
LVEF ≤0.40 (ACE-inhibitor intolerant)	1,700
LVEF ≤0.40	2,500

LVEF = left ventricular ejection fraction
ACE = angiotensin-converting enzyme
CHARM = Candesartan Cilexetil in Heart Failure
Assessment of Reduction in Mortality and Morbidity

CHARM study population is also receiving a β-blocker, the results will help to confirm or refute the subgroup analysis of Val-HeFT, suggesting lack of efficacy (or possibly an adverse effect) when the three drugs are used together. Finally, the preserved systolic function arm of the study represents the first large-scale clinical trial designed to assess the effects of any form of therapy in patients with heart failure on this basis. These results will be extremely welcome, since patients with diastolic dysfunction have been markedly underrepresented in heart failure trials despite the fact that they make up approximately 50% of the heart failure population.

Inhibition of Aldosterone in Heart Failure

Aldosterone 'escape'. Patients with heart failure may have high levels of circulating aldosterone despite treatment with an ACE inhibitor or an ARB, a condition referred to as *aldosterone escape.*[64-66] Aldosterone release from the adrenal gland is influenced by factors other than Ang II.[67] Aldosterone is known to have a variety of effects throughout the body.

Comparison	Results
Candesartan 4 to 32 mg vs placebo (open-label ACE inhibitor in both arms)	Ongoing
Candesartan 4 to 32 mg vs placebo	Ongoing
Candesartan 4 to 32 mg vs placebo (open-label ACE inhibitor allowed)	Ongoing

In the kidney, it promotes salt and water retention, as well as loss of potassium and magnesium. Aldosterone has also been associated with sympathetic stimulation and parasympathetic inhibition, baroreceptor dysfunction, vascular damage, and impaired arterial compliance. In addition, a considerable body of evidence suggests that aldosterone is an important factor in the development of cardiac fibrosis.[68,69] The deposition of fibrous tissue is increased in the failing heart, and the quantity and structure of the ECM component of the myocardium are important determinants of systolic and diastolic function. Thus, it appears that aldosterone may play an important role in the pathogenesis of the deleterious heart remodeling that has been implicated in the progression of cardiac dysfunction. Fibrosis is also believed to be related to the development of ventricular arrhythmias because of the mechanical effects of increased fibrous tissue in disrupting the normal transmission of depolarization throughout the myocardium.

The Randomized Aldactone Evaluation Study. The Randomized Aldactone Evaluation Study (RALES)[70] was or-

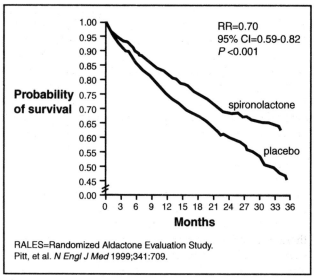

Figure 11: The RALES trial. Effect of spironolactone on survival.

RALES=Randomized Aldactone Evaluation Study.
Pitt, et al. *N Engl J Med* 1999;341:709.

ganized to test the hypothesis that aldosterone plays a role in the pathogenesis of heart failure and to determine if blockade of aldosterone might lead to an improvement in the natural history of patients. The study was designed to assess whether the addition of spironolactone (Aldactone®), an aldosterone-receptor blocker, would improve the clinical course of patients with advanced heart failure. Enrollment into RALES required patients to either have NYHA Class IV symptoms at the time of screening or have recently been in Class IV. The 1,663 patients enrolled were randomized to either low-dose spironolactone (25 to 50 mg q.d.) or placebo in addition to their usual heart failure medications, which in more than 90% included either an ACE inhibitor or an ARB.

As shown in Figure 11, mortality in placebo-treated patients was considerable, a finding that confirmed the severity of heart failure in the RALES population. The addition of spironolactone, however, was associated with a 30% reduction in mortality ($P<0.001$). This reduction was attributed to a lower risk of death from progressive heart failure and sudden death from cardiac causes. Spironolactone also decreased frequency of heart failure-related hospitalizations by 35% ($P<0.001$). Overall, the drug was well tolerated at this dose, with only minimal increases in serum potassium levels in both study groups. There was, however, an 8.5% excess incidence of painful gynecomastia in male patients receiving spironolactone in the RALES trial.

Recommendations for the use of spironolactone in treating heart failure patients. Based on the results of RALES, the use of spironolactone is recommended as adjunctive therapy to other neurohormonal blocking agents in patients with either current or recent NYHA Class IV symptoms of heart failure. In this group, a reduction in the potassium supplement dose is usually undertaken at initiation of spironolactone therapy. However, the extent of the required reduction in potassium is, in the authors' experience, highly variable. Reduction of the dose by a third or by half is a reasonable place to begin, but the impact of the drug (even in patients not receiving supplemental potassium) is unpredictable, pointing out the need to measure potassium blood levels on a regular basis. Thus, it is prudent to obtain a set of serum electrolytes after 1 week of spironolactone therapy. The test should be repeated no more than 2 weeks later and then at regular intervals. In the opinion of many heart failure experts, assessment of serum potassium levels should be performed for the duration of spironolactone therapy, since there are instances when hyperkalemia appears months after drug has been added to the regimen. Patients with milder degrees of heart failure who demonstrate evidence of refractory or difficult-to-treat hypokalemia are also candidates for this therapy. However, the long-term effects of spironolactone on the natural history in patients with milder heart failure is unknown at this time.

References

1. Timmermans PB, Wong PC, Chiu AT, et al: Angiotensin II receptors and angiotensin II receptor antagonists. *Pharmacol Rev* 1993;45:205-251.

2. De Gasparo M, Levens NR, Kambler B, et al: The angiotensin II AT_2 receptor subtype. *Angiotensin Receptors* 1994;95-117.

3. Matsubara H: Pathophysiological role of angiotensin II type 2 receptor in cardiovascular and renal diseases. *Circ Res* 1998;83:1182-1191.

4. Ardaillou R: Angiotensin II receptors. *J Am Soc Nephrol* 1999;10:S30-S39.

5. Dzau VJ: Cardiac renin-angiotensin system. Molecular and functional aspects. *Am J Med* 1988;84:22-27.

6. Lindpaintner K, Ganten D: The cardiac renin-angiotensin system. An appraisal of present experimental and clinical evidence. *Circ Res* 1991;68:905-921.

7. Phillips MI, Speakman EA, Kimura B: Levels of angiotensin and molecular biology of the tissue renin angiotensin systems. *Regulatory Peptides* 1993;43:1-20.

8. Dostal DE, Baker KM: The cardiac renin-angiotensin system: conceptual, or a regulator of cardiac function? *Circ Res* 1999;85:643-650.

9. De Mello WC, Danser AH: Angiotensin II and the heart: on the intracrine renin-angiotensin system. *Hypertension* 2000;35:1183-1188.

10. Wollert KC, Drexler H: The renin-angiotensin system and experimental heart failure. *Cardiol Res* 1999;43:838-849.

11. Urata H, Boehm KD, Philip A, et al: Cellular localization and regional distribution of an angiotensin II-forming chymase in the heart. *J Clin Invest* 1993;91:1269-1281.

12. Husain A: The chymase-angiotensin system in humans. *J Hypertens* 1993;11:1155-1159.

13. Takai S, Jin D, Sakaguchi M, et al: Chymase-dependent angiotensin II formation in human vascular tissue. *Circulation* 1999;100:654-658.

14. Ridker PM, Gaboury CL, Conlin PR, et al: Stimulation of plasminogen activator inhibitor in vivo by infusion of angiotensin II. Evidence of a potential interaction between the renin-angiotensin system and fibrinolytic function. *Circulation* 1993;87:1969-1973.

15. Baker KM, Aceto JF: Angiotensin II stimulation of protein synthesis and cell growth in chick heart cells. *Am J Physiol* 1990;259:H610-H618.

16. Schorb W, Booz GW, Dostal DE, et al: Angiotensin II is mitogenic in neonatal rat cardiac fibroblasts. *Circ Res* 1993;72:1245-1254.

17. Sadoshima J, Izumo S: Molecular characterization of angiotensin II-induced hypertrophy of cardiac myocytes and hyperplasia of cardiac fibroblasts. Critical role of the AT_1 receptor subtype. *Circ Res* 1993;73:413-423.

18. St. John MG, Sharpe N: Left ventricular remodeling after myocardial infarction: pathophysiology and therapy. *Circulation* 2000;101:2981-2988.

19. Gaudron P, Eilles C, Kugler I, et al: Progressive left ventricular dysfunction and remodeling after myocardial infarction: potential mechanisms and early predictors. *Circulation* 1993;87:755-763.

20. Cambien F, Poirier O, Lecerf L, et al: Deletion polymorphism in the gene for angiotensin-converting enzyme is a potent risk factor for myocardial infarction. *Nature* 1992;359:641-644.

21. Raynolds MV, Bristow MR, Bush EW, et al: Angiotensin-converting enzyme DD genotype in patients with ischaemic or idiopathic dilated cardiomyopathy. *Lancet* 1993;342:1073-1075.

22. Leckie BJ: Shuffling the cards: polymorphisms of genes for angiotensin-converting enzyme and angiotensinogen are linked to coronary artery disease and hypertension in man. *Curr Biol* 1993;3:124-126.

23. Corvol P, Soubrier F, Jeunemaitre X: Molecular genetics of the renin-angiotensin-aldosterone system in human hypertension. *Curr Opin Endocrine Diabetes* 1995;2:266-275.

24. Nakai K, Itoh C, Miura Y: Deletion polymorphism of the angiotensin I-converting enzyme gene is associated with serum ACE concentration and increased risk for CAD in the Japanese. *Circulation* 1994;90:2199-2202.

25. Perticone F, Ceravolo R, Cosco C, et al: Deletion polymorphism of angiotensin-converting enzyme gene and left ventricu-

lar hypertrophy in southern Italian patients. *J Am Coll Cardiol* 1997;29:365-369.

26. Andersson B, Sylvén C: The DD genotype of the angiotensin-converting enzyme gene is associated with increased mortality in idiopathic heart failure. *J Am Coll Cardiol* 1996; 28:162-167.

27. Dzau VJ, Colucci WS, Hollenberg NK, et al: Relation of the renin-angiotensin-aldosterone system to clinical state in congestive heart failure. *Circulation* 1981;63:645-651.

28. Hodsman GP, Kohzuki M, Howes LG, et al: Neurohormonal responses to chronic myocardial infarction in rats. *Circulation* 1988;78:376-381.

29. Michel JB, Lattion AL, Salzmann JL, et al: Hormonal and cardiac effects of converting enzyme inhibition in rat myocardial infarction. *Circ Res* 1988;62:641-650.

30. Francis GS, McDonald KM, Cohn JN: Neurohormonal activation in preclinical heart failure: remodeling and the potential for intervention. *Circulation* 1993;87:IV90-IV96.

31. Benedict CR, Johnstone DE, Weiner DH, et al: Relation of neurohormonal activation to clinical variable and degree of ventricular dysfunction: a report from the Registry of Studies of Left Ventricular Dysfunction. The SOLVD Investigators. *J Am Coll Cardiol* 1994;23:1410-1420.

32. Benedict CR, Weiner DH, Johnstone DE, et al: Comparative neurohormonal responses in patients with preserved and impaired left ventricular ejection fraction: results of the Studies of Left Ventricular Dysfunction (SOLVD) registry. The SOLVD Investigators. *J Am Coll Cardiol* 1993;22:146A-153A.

33. Hirsch AT, Talsness CE, Schunkert H, et al: Tissue-specific activation of cardiac angiotensin converting enzyme in experimental heart failure. *Circ Res* 1991;69:475-482.

34. Schunkert H, Dzau VJ, Tang SS, et al: Increased rat cardiac angiotensin converting enzyme activity and mRNA expression in pressure overload left ventricular hypertrophy: effects on coronary resistance, contractility, and relaxation. *J Clin Invest* 1990;86: 1913-1920.

35. Lindpaintner K, Lu W, Niedermajer N, et al: Selective activation of cardiac angiotensinogen gene expression ion post-infarction ventricular remodeling in the rat. *J Mol Cell Cardiol* 1993;25: 133-143.

36.   Nio Y, Matsubara H, Murasawa S, et al: Regulation of gene transcription of angiotensin II receptor subtypes in myocardial infarction. *J Clin Invest* 1995;95:46-54.

37.   Lefroy DC, Wharton J, Crake T, et al: Regional changes in angiotensin II receptor density after experimental myocardial infarction. *J Mol Cell Cardiol* 1996;28:429-440.

38.   Yang BC, Phillips MI, Ambuehl PE, et al: Increase in angiotensin II type 1 receptor expression immediately after ischemia-reperfusion in isolated rat hearts. *Circulation* 1997;96:922-926.

39.   Sun Y, Weber KT: Angiotensin II receptor binding following myocardial infarction in the rat. *Cardiovasc Res* 1994;28:1623-1628.

40.   Peng JF, Gurantz D, Cowling RT, et al: TNF-α alters Ang II-medicated cardiac fibroblast function in favor of fibrosis. *J Cardiol Failure* 2000;6:2-21.

41.   Farhy RD, Ho K, Carretero OA, et al: Kinins mediate the antiproliferative effect of ramipril in rat carotid artery. *Biochem Biophys Res Commun* 1992;182:283-288.

42.   Brunner HR, Laragh JH, Baer L, et al: Essential hypertension: renin and aldosterone, heart attack and stroke. *N Engl J Med* 1972;286:441-449.

43.   Alderman MH, Madhavan SH, Ooi WL, et al: Association of the renin-sodium profile with the risk of myocardial infarction in patients with hypertension. *N Engl J Med* 1991;324:1098-1104.

44.   Yusuf S, Pepine CJ, Garces C, et al: Effect of enalapril on myocardial infarction and unstable angina in patients with low ejection fractions. *Lancet* 1992;340:1173-1178.

45.   Pfeffer MA, Braunwald E, Moyé LA, et al: Effect of captopril on mortality and morbidity in patients with left ventricular dysfunction after myocardial infarction. Results of the survival and ventricular enlargement trial. The SAVE Investigators. *N Engl J Med* 1992;327:669-677.

46.   Yusuf S, Sleight P, Pogue J, et al: Effects of an angiotensin-converting-enzyme inhibitor, ramipril, on cardiovascular events in high-risk patients. *N Engl J Med* 2000;342:145-153.

47.   Kober L, Torp-Pedersen C, Carlsen JE, et al: A clinical trial of the angiotensin-converting-enzyme inhibitor trandolapril in patients with left ventricular dysfunction after myocardial infarction. *N Engl J Med* 1995;333:1670-1676.

48. Ambrosioni E, Borghi C, Magnani B: The effect of the angiotensin-converting-enzyme inhibitor zofenopril on mortality and morbidity after anterior myocardial infarction. The Survival of Myocardial Infarction Long-Term Evaluation (SMILE) Study Investigators. *N Engl J Med* 1995;332:80-85.

49. Latini R, Maggioni AP, Flather M, et al: ACE inhibitor use in patients with myocardial infarction. Summary of evidence from clincial trials. *Circulation* 1995;92:3132-3137.

50. Franzosi MG, Santoro E, Zuanetti G, et al: Indications for ACE inhibitors in the early treatment of acute myocardial infarction: systematic overview of individual data from 100,000 patients in randomized trials. *Circulation* 1998;97:2202-2212.

51. Flather MD, Yusuf S, Kober L, et al: Long-term ACE-inhibitor therapy in patients with heart failure or left-ventricular dysfunction: a systematic overview of data from individual patients. ACE-Inhibitor Myocardial Infarction Collaborative Group. *Lancet* 2000;355:1575-1581.

52. Effect of ramipril on mortality and morbidity of survivors of acute myocardial infarction with evidence of heart failure. The Acute Infarction Ramipril Efficacy (AIRE) Study Investigators. *Lancet* 1993;342:821-828.

53. Yusuf S, Pitt B, Davis CE, et al: Effect of enalapril on mortality and the development of heart failure in asymptomatic patients with reduced left ventricular ejection fractions. *N Engl J Med* 1992;327:685-691.

54. Effect of enalapril on survival in patients with reduced left ventricular ejection fractions and congestive heart failure. The SOLVD Investigators. *N Engl J Med* 1991;325:293-302.

55. Greenberg B, Quinones MA, Koilpillai C, et al: Effects of long-term enalapril therapy on cardiac structure and function in patients with left ventricular dysfunction. Results of the SOLVD echocardiography substudy. *Circulation* 1995;91:2573-2581.

56. Effects of enalapril on mortality in severe congestive heart failure. Results of the Cooperative North Scandinavian Enalapril Survival Study (CONSENSUS). The CONSENSUS Trial Study Group. *N Engl J Med* 1987;316:1429-1435.

57. Pitt B, Chang P, Timmermans PB: Angiotensin II receptor antagonists in heart failure: rationale and design of the evaluation of losartan in the elderly (ELITE) trial. *Cardiovasc Drugs Ther* 1995;9:693-700.

58. Goodfriend TL, Elliot ME, Catt KJ: Angiotensin receptors and their antagonists. *N Engl J Med* 1996;334:1649-1654.

59. Grafe M, Bossaller C, Graf K, et al: Effect of angiotensin-converting-enzyme inhibition on bradykinin metabolism by vascular endothelial cells. *Am J Physiol* 1993;264:H1493-H1497.

60. Cheng CP, Onishi K, Ohte N, et al: Functional effects of endogenous bradykinin in congestive heart failure. *J Am Coll Cardiol* 1998;31:1679-1686.

61. Pitt B, Poole-Wilson PA, Segal R, et al: Effect of losartan compared with captopril on mortality in patients with symptomatic heart failure: randomized trial—the Losartan Heart Failure Survival Study ELITE II. *Lancet* 2000;355:1582-1587.

62. Pitt B, Segal R, Martinez FA, et al: Randomised trial of losartan versus captopril in patients over 65 with heart failure (Evaluation of Losartan in the Elderly Study, ELITE). *Lancet* 1997;349:747-752.

63. McKelvie RS, Yusuf S, Pericak D, et al: Comparison of candesartan, enalapril, and their combination in congestive heart failure: randomized evaluation of strategies for left ventricular dysfunction (RESOLVD) pilot study. The RESOLVD Pilot Study Investigators. *Circulation* 1999;100:1056-1064.

64. Staessen J, Lijnen P, Fagard R, et al: Rise in plasma concentration of aldosterone during long-term angiotensin II suppression. *J Endocrinol* 1981;91:457-465.

65. Borghi C, Boschi S, Ambrosioni E, et al: Evidence of a partial escape of renin-angiotensin-aldosterone blockade in patients with acute myocardial infarction treated with ACE inhibitors. *J Clin Pharmacol* 1993;33:40-45.

66. Cleland JG, Dargie HJ, Hodsman GP, et al: Captopril in heart failure. A double blind controlled trial. *Br Heart J* 1984;52:530-535.

67. Okubo S, Niimura F, Nishimura H, et al. Angiotensin-independent mechanism for aldosterone synthesis during chronic extracellular fluid volume depletion. *J Clin Invest* 1997;99:855-860.

68. Brilla CG, Rupp H, Funck R, et al: The renin-angiotensin-aldosterone system and myocardial collagen matrix remodelling in congestive heart failure. *Eur Heart J* 1995;16:107-109.

69. Weber KT: Extracellular matrix remodeling in heart failure: a role for de novo angiotensin II generation. *Circulation* 1997; 96:4065-4082.

70. Pitt B, Zannad F, Remme WJ, et al: The effect of spironolactone on morbidity and mortality in patients with severe heart failure. Randomized Aldactone Evaluation Study Investigators. *N Engl J Med* 1999;341:709-717.

Chapter 5

β-Blocker Therapy

Those physicians who completed their training before the new millennium have had the opportunity to witness a remarkable turn of events regarding the use of β-blockers in patients with heart failure. Once contraindicated out of fear of further compromising cardiac function, β-blockers have been clearly shown to substantially improve cardiac function and the overall clinical course of heart failure patients. So strong is the evidence that has emerged in support of β-blocker use in heart failure patients that, along with angiotensin-converting enzyme (ACE) inhibitors and diuretics (in patients who are fluid overloaded), β-blockers are now considered to be a standard therapy for treatment of heart failure in this population.[1] This chapter reviews the rationale for the use of β-blockers in heart failure patients, the relevant clinical trials that support their widespread use, and the practical aspects of β-blocker treatment, such as initiation, up-titration, and management of side effects.

Why Are β-Blockers So Effective?

In the patient with impaired left ventricular (LV) systolic function, a variety of local and systemic responses are activated to compensate for a reduction in cardiac output and/or arterial perfusion pressure. Researchers now recognize that although many of these compensatory mechanisms provide important support of cardiac function, they are better

Table 1: Adverse Consequences of Norepinephrine

- Peripheral vasoconstriction
- Salt and water retention
- Increased release of renin activity from the kidney
- Down-regulation of β-adrenergic receptors
- Arrhythmogenesis
- Myocyte toxicity
- Myocyte hypertrophy
- Fibroblast production of extracellular matrix

suited for short-term protection than for long-term maintenance (eg, the activation of the sympathetic nervous system).[2,3] Catecholamine-mediated increases in heart rate, myocardial contractility, and peripheral vascular tone are ideally suited for acute events, such as dehydration or blood loss, that threaten the viability of the organism. However, when maintained over an extended period in patients with chronic cardiac dysfunction, the effects of catecholamines are now recognized to be highly deleterious. The adverse consequences of increased sympathetic nervous system activity in heart failure are summarized in Table 1. Catecholamines increase vasomotor tone and salt and water retention both directly and by stimulating release of renin activity from the kidney. This increase in plasma renin leads to increases in angiotensin II levels, which promote salt and water retention and peripheral vasoconstriction—effects that lead to worsening heart failure. The resultant increase in wall stress caused by elevated intracardiac pressures and volumes further worsens cardiac function by increasing the load on the failing heart. Down-regulation and desensitization of β-adrenergic receptors in the heart[4] and throughout the body in response to high catecholamine levels compromise the organism's ability to respond to stress by blunting the 'fight or flight' response.

Catecholamines are known to be highly arrhythmogenic and play an important role in the development of atrial and potentially lethal ventricular arrhythmias in heart failure patients. Exposure of cardiac cells to catecholamines reduces cell viability[5] through direct toxicity and by inducing programmed cell death (apoptosis). Evidence also confirms that catecholamines have potentially harmful effects on cardiac structure that are related to stimulation of myocyte hypertrophy and fibroblast production of extracellular matrix (ECM) proteins. These cellular effects play an important role in promoting cardiac remodeling, a process critical to the development of progressive cardiac dysfunction.[6] The theoretical basis for the use of β-blockers in heart failure patients is based on the observation that they protect the heart from these long-term harmful effects of catecholamines.

Activation of the Sympathetic Nervous System in Patients with Cardiac Dysfunction

Neurohormonal activation occurs early in the setting of LV systolic dysfunction, and there is evidence that it may precede the onset of heart failure. The Studies of Left Ventricular Dysfunction (SOLVD) trial sampled neurohormone levels in plasma from a subset of patients who were included in the clinical trials.[7] The results showed that patients with asymptomatic LV dysfunction (ie, left ventricular ejection fraction [LVEF] <0.35 but no symptoms or treatment prescribed for heart failure) had evidence of significant elevations in plasma norepinephrine levels compared to an age- and sex-matched control group (Figure 1). The patients with low EF who either had symptoms of heart failure or were receiving therapy for heart failure had even higher plasma norepinephrine levels than the asymptom-

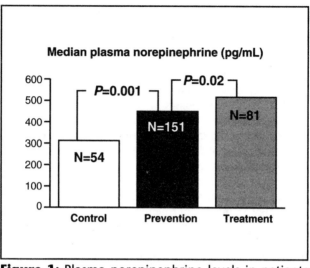

Figure 1: Plasma norepinephrine levels in patients with LV dysfunction. These data from the Studies of Left Ventricular Dysfunction (SOLVD) trial depict mean plasma norepinephrine levels in a subset of patients enrolled in the prevention and treatment arms of the study and in a group of age- and sex-matched controls. Patients were sampled before randomization to study drug (ie, enalapril or placebo). All patients had evidence of LV dysfunction with EF <0.35. Despite the fact that patients in the prevention arm were asymptomatic, there was still evidence of activation of the sympathetic nervous system, as indicated by the significant increase in the level of norepinephrine. Symptomatic patients had even higher levels, indicating further activation as the condition progresses. (Adapted from Francis GS, Benedict C, Johnstone DE, et al: Comparison of neuroendocrine activation in patients with left ventricular dysfunction with and without congestive heart failure. A substudy of the Studies of Left Ventricular Dysfunction (SOLVD). *Circulation* 1990;82:1724-1729.)

atic patients. This early increase in plasma norepinephrine develops in response to a fall in cardiac output and/or arterial perfusion pressure.[8] In the short term, it helps to maintain perfusion of vital organs. However, as heart failure progresses and patients become more symptomatic, there are further increases in catecholamine levels in an effort to maintain circulatory homeostasis. Powerful evidence that these increases in circulating catecholamines are not favorable comes from the multiple surveys that demonstrate plasma norepinephrine to be a strong and highly independent predictor of the clinical course of heart failure patients.[9,10] In these surveys, the higher the level of circulating catecholamines, the worse the prognosis.

The Emergence of β-Blocker Therapy in Treating Heart Failure Patients

Although the rationale for using β-blockers now seems logical and even intuitive, most of the harmful effects of catecholamines were not clearly defined or recognized 30 years ago when β-blockers were first initiated in heart failure patients. What was widely appreciated at that time was that administration of β-blockers to a patient with LV dysfunction could precipitate worsening heart failure. While this is certainly true, the likelihood of causing a patient's condition to deteriorate can be greatly diminished by using β-blocking drugs in a judicious fashion, including avoiding administration to patients who are acutely decompensated or who have evidence of volume overload. Even more important is the recognition that problems can be successfully avoided in most patients by initiating therapy at a low dose and gradually up-titrating the β-blocker over time. In fact, recent clinical trials with β-blockers have found these agents are very well tolerated, even in patients with advanced heart failure.

Initial uncontrolled studies in heart failure patients and retrospective analyses of studies that evaluated subgroups of myocardial infarction (MI) survivors with heart failure yielded surprisingly (at the time) positive results for the use of β-blockers in these populations.[11-13] Gradually, these initial encouraging results began to stimulate more widespread interest in the somewhat 'heretical' notion that β-blockers could not only be safely given to heart failure patients, but also might substantially improve patients' clinical course. During the 1980s and early 1990s, several small controlled trials showed that the long-term administration of β-blockers was associated with improvement in the clinical status of heart failure patients.[14-20] Although LVEF is initially slightly reduced when β-blockers are first administered,[18] there was convincing evidence that maintenance of therapy over several months resulted in a significant (and often dramatic) improvement in cardiac function. Moreover, these patients also experienced improvement in their clinical status, as evidenced by their movement to a lower, more favorable New York Heart Association (NYHA) class.

Interestingly, some of the impetus for the further development of β-blockers in heart failure came from an unexpected quarter. When evidence that β-blocking drugs might favorably affect the clinical course of heart failure patients first emerged, it became increasingly apparent that the long-term effects of inotropic stimulation of the heart were harmful. The Prospective Randomized Milrinone Survival Evaluation (PROMISE) study showed that the use of oral milrinone, a phosphodiesterase inhibitor, was associated with increased mortality in heart failure patients.[21] Dose-dependent increases in mortality were also seen with the inotropic agent vesnarinone in patients with advanced heart failure.[22] Perhaps even more important was evidence that xamoterol (Corwin®), a β-blocking drug with intrinsic sympathomimetic activity (ISA), also increased mortality.[23] Thus, stimulation of the adrenergic pathway, either at the level of the receptor or farther down the signaling cascade, appeared to adversely affect heart failure patients. These results raised the possibility that the opposite approach (blocking the β-adrenergic receptor) might be beneficial in improving the clinical course of heart failure patients.

Results from more ambitious clinical trials assessing the long-term effects of β-blockers played an important role in moving the field forward. However, the initial placebo-controlled trials that included clinically relevant end points, such as the Metoprolol in Dilated Cardiomyopathy (MDC) study[24] and Cardiac Insufficiency Bisoprolol Study I (CIBIS-I),[25] failed to provide convincing evidence of efficacy. Nonetheless, there was a promising reduction, though of borderline statistical significance, in the combined end point of death and need for cardiac transplantation in patients who received metoprolol in the MDC study. Additionally, there was a trend toward a reduction in all-cause mortality in favor of the bisoprolol (Zebeta®)-treated group in CIBIS-I. Though by no means definitive, the results of these relatively small and underpowered studies were highly promising. They also served the important function of drawing attention to the possibility that β-blockers might indeed be useful in treating heart failure patients, and they provided a platform on which the larger studies that eventually proved the 'β-blocker hypothesis' could be constructed.

Evidence Supporting the Use of β-Blockers in Heart Failure Patients

The sine qua non for efficacy of any treatment in chronic heart failure is that the approach being evaluated (drug, device, or management strategy) is shown to have a favorable effect on a clinically relevant end point in well-designed, placebo-controlled clinical trials. For example, the acceptance of ACE inhibitors as a standard therapy in heart failure is based on evidence from controlled clinical trials such as the Cooperative North Scandinavian Enalapril Survival Study (CONSENSUS)[26]

Table 2: Recent Trials of β-Blockers in Heart Failure

Trial	Size (n)	Drug
US Carvedilol Trials	1,094	carvedilol (Coreg®)
CIBIS-II	2,647	bisoprolol (Zebeta®)
MERIT-HF	3,991	metoprolol CR/XL (Toprol-XL®)
BEST	2,708	bucindolol (Bextra®)
COPERNICUS	2,289	carvedilol

EF = ejection fraction
NYHA = New York Heart Association
CIBIS = Cardiac Insufficiency Bisoprolol Study
MERIT-HF = Metoprolol Randomized Intervention Trial in Heart Failure

and SOLVD.[27,28] These studies demonstrated that ACE inhibitors improve survival, reduce hospitalization rates, and have other favorable effects compared to standard therapy. The results of the Veterans Administration Heart Failure Trial (V-HeFT-II) that demonstrated a favorable effect of enalapril (Vasotec®) on mortality compared to the vasodilator combination of hydralazine and isosorbide dinitrate (Hyd/Iso) provided evidence that these effects were not simply a result of the vasodilating properties of ACE inhibitors.[29]

To date, at least five well-designed, large-scale trials (>1,000 patients) have evaluated the effects of β-blockers in

Target Dose	EF for Entry	NYHA Class
25 mg b.i.d. (50 mg b.i.d. if weight ≥85 kg)	≤0.35	II-IV (mostly II-III)
10 mg q.d.	≤0.35	III-IV (mostly III)
200 mg q.d.	≤0.35	II-IV (mostly II-III)
100 mg b.i.d.	≤0.35	III-IV
25 mg b.i.d.	≤0.25	III-IV

BEST = β-Blocker Evaluation of Survival Trial
COPERNICUS = Carvedilol Prospective Randomized Cumulative Survival

heart failure (Table 2).[30-34] All of these trials used a double-blinded, placebo-controlled design to evaluate the effects of a β-blocker in patients with chronic heart failure caused by LV systolic dysfunction. Patients included in the trials were already receiving standard therapy that, in most cases, included an ACE inhibitor or angiotensin-receptor blocker (ARB). Thus, the studies evaluated the effects of combined β-blocker and ACE inhibitor therapy with the effects of ACE inhibitor therapy alone. Although NYHA class varied between the studies, the patients included were generally stable

Table 3: Results of β-Blocker Trials

Trial	Drug
US Carvedilol Trials	carvedilol (Coreg®)
CIBIS-II	bisoprolol (Zebeta®)
MERIT-HF	metoprolol CR/XL (Toprol-XL®)
BEST	bucindolol (Bextra®)
COPERNICUS	carvedilol

* Annualized from 6 months.
** Mortality was not a primary end point.
*** Reduction in mortality in BEST was not significant.

and free of fluid overload at the time of randomization to β-blocker or placebo.

Table 3 summarizes the results of the β-blocker trials. Interestingly, none of these trials was allowed to run to completion. In each case, the data safety monitoring board (DSMB) that was responsible for overseeing the study recommended premature termination. In all of the studies, except for the β-blocker Evaluation of Survival Trial (BEST), this decision was based on the overwhelmingly positive results, including highly significant reductions in mortality, with the β-blocker compared to placebo.

The US Carvedilol Trials program was a series of four independent trials with similar entry criteria and common procedures.[30] All four trials were double-blinded, placebo-controlled studies that compared the effects of carvedilol (Coreg®) to those of placebo. Although patients were assigned to these trials based on their performance on a 6-minute walk test, it was the intention of the investigators to use pooled data from the trials to assess issues such as the

Annual Placebo Mortality	Mortality Risk Reduction
12%*	65%**
13%	34%
11%	34%
17%	10%***
19%	35%

effects of therapy on survival and the tolerability of carvedilol in heart failure. The US Carvedilol Trials program was stopped when it became apparent that patients randomized to carvedilol were doing considerably better than those assigned to placebo. There was a 65% reduction (P <0.001) in all-cause mortality in the carvedilol-treated patients, all-cause hospitalization was reduced by 29%, and there were important reductions in cardiovascular and heart failure hospitalizations in the study population. As shown in Figure 2, combined risk of death or hospitalization was reduced by 38% (P <0.01). LVEF was significantly increased in the carvedilol group compared to the placebo group, and there were improvements in the quality-of-life scores and in NYHA class associated with carvedilol treatment. Overall, tolerability of the drug was good, with no significant increase in the percentage of patients who stopped taking carvedilol compared to the percentage who stopped taking placebo during the course of the trial.

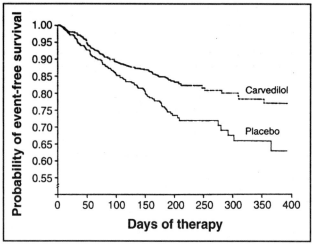

Figure 2: Probability of combined risk of death or hospitalization in the US Carvedilol Trials program. Overall, there was a 38% reduction in carvedilol-treated patients (*P* ≤0.001). (Adapted from Packer M, Bristow MR, Cohn JN, et al: The effect of carvedilol on morbidity and mortality in patients with chronic heart failure. US Carvedilol Heart Failure Study Group. *N Engl J Med* 1996;334:1349-1355.)

The Multicenter Oral Carvedilol Heart Failure Assessment (MOCHA) study was one of the components in the US Carvedilol Trials program.[35] It was designed to obtain information about the dose-response effects of carvedilol. In MOCHA, patients were randomly assigned to groups in which carvedilol was titrated to a maximum dose of either 6.25 mg, 12.5 mg, or 25 mg twice daily. There was also a placebo control group. The results (Figure 3) show a significant association between the dose of carvedilol and the increase in EF that occurred over a 6-month follow-up. Interestingly, even the lowest dose of carvedilol tested in this study, 6.25 mg twice daily, was associated with a statistically significant increase in EF compared to placebo. The

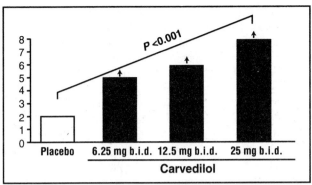

Figure 3: Changes in LVEF over time in patients on carvedilol. The patients on carvedilol (n=261) and placebo (n=84) had EF measured by radioisotope angiogram before and after 6 months of therapy in the Multicenter Oral Carvedilol Heart Failure Assessment (MOCHA) trial. The results show that there is a dose-related increase in LVEF with carvedilol. However, even at a dose of 6.25 mg b.i.d., there was a significant increase in EF over time compared to placebo. (Adapted from Bristow MR, Gilbert EM, Abraham WT, et al: Carvedilol produces dose-related improvements in left ventricular function and survival in subjects with chronic heart failure. MOCHA Investigators. *Circulation* 1996;94:2807-2816.)

changes seen in EF were roughly paralleled by reductions in hospitalization rate and survival. Although patients on the 25-mg dose demonstrated the greatest benefits of therapy for these end points, those receiving the 6.25-mg dose also did significantly better than their placebo control counterparts. When applied to clinical practice, these results indicate that an attempt should be made to increase carvedilol to the recommended maximal dose. However, it is reassuring that patients who are able to tolerate lower doses (ie, 6.25 mg and 12.5 mg twice daily) are also likely to receive considerable benefit from this therapy.

In the Cardiac Insufficiency Bisoprolol Study-II (CIBIS-II), the effects of bisoprolol (Zebeta®) were compared to placebo in patients with NYHA Class III-IV heart failure.[31] However, the mortality seen in the placebo group (13%) suggested that the population was probably a mixture of NYHA Class II-III, rather than patients in Class IV (more advanced disease). As in the other large β-blocker trials, the drug was tested in the context of background therapy that included an ACE inhibitor. The results showed that bisoprolol was highly effective in improving the clinical course of the patients studied. There was a highly significant 34% reduction ($P < 0.0001$) in all-cause mortality (the primary end point of CIBIS-II) in patients receiving the β-blocker, which was largely caused by a 44% reduction in sudden death ($P = 0.011$). Unlike the results from the smaller CIBIS-I trial that suggested a more favorable effect in patients with a nonischemic etiology, the findings from CIBIS-II did not show any significant interaction between etiology of heart failure and efficacy of bisoprolol.

The Metoprolol CR/XL Randomized Intervention Trial in Congestive Heart Failure (MERIT-HF) evaluated the effects of metoprolol CR/XL (Toprol-XL®), the long-acting form of metoprolol, in patients with NYHA Class II-IV heart failure symptoms. Most patients were Class II-III, however, and there were several of the more severely symptomatic patients in the study. The 3,991 patients in MERIT-HF were randomly assigned to receive either placebo or metoprolol CR/XL in addition to standard therapy that, in almost all cases, included an ACE inhibitor or an ARB. The dose of β-blocker was initiated at 25 mg (12.5 mg in more severely symptomatic patients) and up-titrated gradually to a target dose of 200 mg daily. The actual dose of metoprolol CR/XL averaged 159 mg, and 64% of participants achieved the target dose of the drug, indicating how well this therapy was tolerated in the heart failure population. Over the course of MERIT-HF, 14% of metoprolol

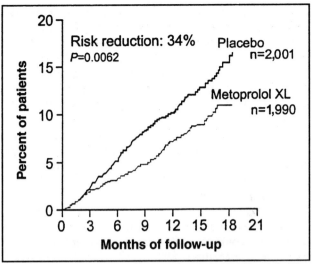

Figure 4: Total mortality in the MERIT-HF trial. The benefits of metoprolol XL begin to appear approximately 3 months after the initiation of therapy, and they increase over time. (Adapted from Effect of metoprolol CR/XL in chronic heart failure: Metoprolol CR/XL Randomized Intervention Trial in Congestive Heart Failure (MERIT-HF). *Lancet* 1999;353:2001-2007).

CR/XL-treated patients and 15.5% of placebo-treated patients required permanent discontinuation of study. These results reinforce the fact that β-blockers, such as metoprolol CR/XL, are well tolerated when they are initiated at a low dose and gradually up-titrated in appropriate patients. The primary end point of MERIT-HF was all-cause mortality, which was reduced by 34% (P=0.0062) with metoprolol CR/XL compared to placebo (Figure 4). In patients with NYHA Class II-III symptoms, death was usually sudden (presumably on the basis of lethal ventricular arrhythmias). Death caused by worsening pump failure occurred in only a minority of patients. Since most patients with heart failure fall within these classes, the effect of metoprolol CR/XL on sudden cardiac death is of considerable importance. The results of MERIT-HF showed that β-blockade resulted in a highly significant 41% (P=0.0002) reduction in sudden death. Mortality caused by progressive pump failure was also significantly reduced in patients who received metoprolol CR/XL, as were all-cause, cardiovascular, and heart failure hospitalizations.

The three studies described conclusively showed that β-blocker therapy substantially improves the clinical course of patients with NYHA Class II-III symptoms of heart failure. However, whether β-blockers can be safely given to patients with more advanced symptoms and whether this type of therapy improves survival in such patients was not adequately addressed, since these studies included only a small minority of patients with more advanced heart failure.

Two recent studies have assessed the effects of β-blockers in more severely ill patients. However, although BEST and the Carvedilol Prospective Randomized Cumulative Survival (COPERNICUS) study did include more severely ill heart failure patients, these patients were considered by the investigators to be clinically stable at the time of randomization. For example, in COPERNICUS, hospitalized patients receiving intravenous (IV) diuretics could still be enrolled. However, patients were expected to have no evidence of fluid overload, and they were required to be off inotropic agents, such as dobutamine or milrinone, and IV vasodilators, such as nitroglycerin or nitroprusside, at least 4 days before beginning the study. Nonetheless, based on the mean EF in the patients at the time of entry into the study and the observed mortality in the placebo groups in both trials, it is clear that these patients were sicker than those in the other β-blocker heart failure trials.

In BEST, patients were randomized to bucindolol (Bextra®) or to placebo in addition to their standard heart failure medications.[33] The DSMB recommended stopping the trial based on the fact that the reduction in all-cause mortality with bucindolol was only about 10%. While trending toward a favorable effect of bucindolol, these results did not achieve statistical significance. Whether the lesser reduction in mortality with bucindolol compared with other agents was related to the properties of the drug or to the characteristics of the BEST population (or to a combination of these two factors) will likely never be fully known. The BEST study included more severely ill patients than did previous studies, and it included substantially higher percentages of African-American patients, women, and veterans than previous β-blocker studies. Subgroup analysis of the NYHA Class IV and African-American patients showed that these populations, in particular, fared poorly with bucindolol therapy. However, the pharmacologic profile of bucindolol is somewhat different than that of the other agents, which also may have contributed to the only moderate beneficial effects seen in BEST. Bucindolol-treated patients experienced a significant reduction in plasma norepinephrine levels, presumably on the basis of the β_2-blocking properties of the drug that resulted in presynaptic inhibition of catecholamine release. It is possible that in selected patients with more severe heart failure, this reduction in catecholamines further worsened already tenuous cardiac function and, as a result, the clinical condition deteriorated. An adverse outcome in these patients would then offset and moderate a more favorable effect in less severely compromised patients who benefited from bucindolol.

In contrast, the results of the COPERNICUS study demonstrate that at least some β-blockers are well tolerated and highly effective in treating patients with more advanced heart failure.[34] The entry criteria for COPERNICUS are outlined in Table 4. That the COPERNICUS population enrolled more severely ill patients than the US Carvedilol Trials program, CIBIS-II, and MERIT-HF is strongly sug-

Table 4: Entry Criteria for COPERNICUS

- Etiology of heart failure could be ischemic or nonischemic
- LVEF <25%
- Symptoms of heart failure at rest or with minimal exertion continuously for at least 2 months
- On therapy for heart failure, including diuretics and an ACE inhibitor (with or without digoxin)
- Diuretics adjusted so that patients were euvolemic
- Intravenous (IV) diuretics permitted, but use of IV vasodilators or inotropic agents within 4 days excluded

gested by patients' lower EF on entry and by the 18.7% annual mortality in the placebo group in COPERNICUS. In this study, patients were assigned to either carvedilol or placebo in addition to their usual therapy. As shown in Figure 5a, at the time when the study was prematurely stopped by the DSMB, the carvedilol-treated patients had a 35% reduction in all-cause mortality (P <0.00013), the primary end point of the study. The reduction in mortality rates was observed in all prespecified patient subgroups, including those based on age, gender, EF higher or lower than 30%, heart failure hospitalization within 1 year, and location within or outside of North America. Carvedilol also reduced the secondary end point of death or cardiovascular hospitalization by 27% (P <0.00002). Perhaps as impressive as the improvement in survival was the excellent tolerability of carvedilol in this population (Figure 5b). The results show that after 12 months of therapy, 13% of patients treated with carvedilol required withdrawal from therapy compared to 15% in the placebo group (P=0.02). The finding in COPERNICUS that even patients

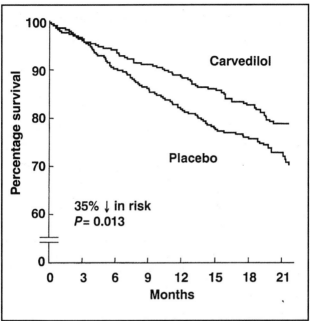

Figure 5a: Efficacy and tolerability of carvedilol in patients with advanced heart failure. These data are from the COPERNICUS study, which included patients who were symptomatic at rest or with minimal exercise for more than 2 months and LVEF <0.25. This panel depicts the life table curves for patients randomized to carvedilol and those who received placebo. Carvedilol-treated patients experienced a highly significant 35% reduction in all-cause mortality, the primary end point of this study.

with advanced (albeit stable) heart failure could tolerate the initiation and maintenance of carvedilol therapy is extremely important, since it provides reassurance about the tolerability of β-blockers in patients with less advanced heart failure.

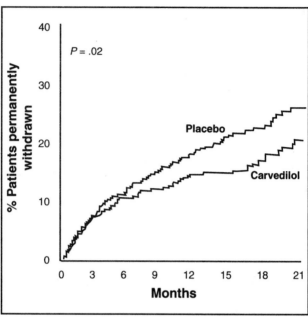

Figure 5b: This panel depicts the curves for discontinuation of the study drug in COPERNICUS. The results demonstrate the excellent tolerability of the β-blocker even in this population with advanced heart failure. (Adapted from Packer M, Coats AJ, Fowler MB, et al: Effect of carvedilol on survival in severe chronic heart failure. *N Engl J Med* 2001;344:1651-1658.)

Which β-Blockers Should Be Used to Treat Heart Failure?

Based on the results of the studies described above, there should be no doubt about the potential for improvement in patients treated with β-blockers. However, the β-blockers that are now available are not a homogeneous group of drugs. A classification of β-blockers based on their pharmacologic properties is shown in Table 5. The differences between drugs are based on whether they are selective for the β_1-adrenergic receptor, as opposed to providing nonselective blockade of β_1 and β_2 subtypes. Further differentiation is based on whether a particular agent has additional properties, such as α_1-adrenergic blocking properties (that would protect against α_1 stimulation of cardiac cells as well as block α_1-mediated peripheral vasoconstriction) or other vasodilating or antioxidant effects.

The pharmacokinetics of the drugs may also influence their efficacy in heart failure. The clinical relevance of such differences is shown by the poor initial tolerability of propranolol (Inderal®).[36] This agent depresses contractile function[37] and causes acutely unfavorable hemodynamic effects, including increased systemic vascular resistance, increased pulmonary artery wedge pressure, and reduced cardiac output. These effects are based on the fact that propranolol is a nonselective β-blocker that lacks additional properties to counteract the blockade of β_1 and β_2 receptors. As a result, it confers more extensive inhibition of the adrenergic system than a β_1-selective agent such as metoprolol. Researchers believe that the greater magnitude of adrenergic blockade in the absence of any additional favorable properties to help offset the loss of inotropic support is the cause of the hemodynamic and clinical decompensation seen with propranolol. Carvedilol is also a nonselective β-blocker, but it has additional α_1-blocking effects that produce vasodilation. This helps unload the heart when the inotropic support, which is mediated through the β_1 and β_2 receptors, is blocked. Consequently, carvedilol is well tolerated, even in patients with advanced heart failure, as was noted in the COPERNICUS study. Based on these considerations, clinicians can conclude that only drugs that have been shown to be effective in large-scale clinical trials (ie, carvedilol, metoprolol CR/XL, and bisoprolol) should be used in treating heart failure patients. Recommendations regarding the use of other drugs must await the results from studies assessing their tolerability and efficacy in the heart failure population.

Table 5: Classification of β-Blockers

Drug	β₁ Blockade	β₂ Blockade
propranolol (Inderal®)	+	+
metoprolol (Toprol-XL®)	+	−
bisoprolol (Zebeta®)	+	−
bucindolol (Bextra®)	+	+
carvedilol (Coreg®)	+	+

When to Use β-Blockers in Heart Failure Patients

The use of β-blockers in treating patients with heart failure is now well established. A recently published 'white paper' by the Care Standards Committee of the Heart Failure Society of America (HFSA) positions β-blocker therapy as standard treatment for heart failure patients.[38] The HFSA recommendations conclude that "β-blocker therapy should be routinely administered to clinically stable patients with LV systolic dysfunction (LVEF ≤40%) and mild to moderate heart failure symptoms (ie, NYHA Class II-III) who are on standard therapy, which typically includes ACE inhibitors, diuretics as needed to control fluid retention, and digoxin." Thus, β-blocker therapy has come full circle. What was once strongly contraindicated is now considered to be a cornerstone of the therapeutic approach to treating heart failure patients!

Now, β-blockers are recommended for treatment of symptomatic NYHA Class II-III patients who have heart failure on the basis of LV systolic dysfunction. Patients should be euvolemic at the time of treatment initiation because patients who are clearly fluid overloaded have a greater likelihood of having an adverse effect, even when low doses of β-blocker are used. Most heart failure pa-

α_1 Blockade	Vasodilation	Other Properties
–	–	–
–	–	–
–	–	–
Mild	+	–
+	+	Antioxidant

tients show evidence of volume overload, and many have symptoms at rest (eg, Class IV) at some time during the course of their illness. This should not be viewed as an absolute contraindication to β-blocker use, but simply as a sign that such therapy should be temporarily deferred. Initiation of β-blocker therapy should not be attempted until patients are diuresed and stabilized. β-blocker therapy should never be used as 'bail-out' therapy for patients who present in an acutely decompensated state, since the benefits manifest only over time. The initial blockade of β-adrenergic support may cause considerable worsening in poorly compensated patients and in those with evidence of volume overload, since such patients may have no margin of reserve to accommodate even a small and temporary decrement in cardiac function.

Recent evidence from the COPERNICUS study also suggests that β-blockers (in this case, carvedilol) are well tolerated and effective in reducing mortality in patients with more advanced heart failure.[34] Patients in COPERNICUS had symptoms at rest or with minimal exercise for a period of 2 months or more despite receiving optimal medical management, including, in most cases, an ACE inhibitor or ARB. Patients randomized to carvedilol had a 35% reduction in all-cause mortality, the primary end point in

COPERNICUS. In keeping with the COPERNICUS entry criteria, patients with more advanced heart failure who are being considered for β-blocker therapy should be euvolemic at the time of therapy initiation. Additionally, although they can be hospitalized and receiving IV diuretics at the time of therapy initiation, patients should have been off IV inotropic agents or vasodilators for at least 4 days.

Some experts have had success initiating and maintaining β-blockers in patients with even more severe heart failure who require IV inotropic therapy. In these cases, the β-blocker is initiated while the patient is in the hospital and under careful observation for evidence of further compromise of his or her already tenuous state. Since β-agonists, such as dobutamine, compete with the β-blocker for β-receptor occupancy, β-blocker therapy is usually initiated using milrinone, a phosphodiesterase inhibitor, to provide inotropic support. The effects of milrinone are not inhibited by the concomitant administration of a β-blocker, since this drug bypasses the β-receptor and improves contractility by blocking the breakdown of cyclic adenosine monophosphate (cAMP). In our experience, initiation of β-blocker therapy in this population can, in many cases, improve cardiac function to the extent that inotropic therapy can be discontinued over time. However, the use of β-blockers in patients who require inotropic therapy remains investigational, and such therapy should be administered only by heart failure specialists who are experienced in this area.

Use of β-Blockers in Asymptomatic Patients

At present, little data exist that describe the efficacy of β-blocker therapy in patients with asymptomatic (ie, NYHA Class I) LV dysfunction. However, a strong case can be made for using β-blockers in such patients, based on the fact that early activation of the sympathetic nervous system is involved in the progression of heart failure[4] and on data from limited, but generally promising, studies that incorporated asymptomatic patients. The Australia-New Zealand (ANZ) study evaluated the long-term effects of β-blockers in patients with cardiac dysfunction caused by underlying ischemic disease.[39] Approximately 30% of the population was asymptomatic at the time of randomization to either carvedilol or placebo. For the two primary end points of the study, carvedilol significantly increased the LVEF but had no significant effect on exercise performance. The results showed that carvedilol was associated with a 26% reduction (P=0.02) in disease progression, a combined end point consisting of mortality, hospitalizations, and sustained requirement for an increase in heart failure medication. There was also evidence that patients treated with carvedilol experienced a reduction in LV volume, a phenomenon termed *reverse remodeling*. Since adverse LV remodeling plays a critical role in the progressive deterioration in cardiac function, such improvements in cardiac structure are believed to be related to the clinical benefits of β-blocker therapy.

β-Blocker Therapy in the Post-MI Patient

Although β-blockers have been shown to reduce reinfarction rates and increase survival post-MI, most studies were performed in an earlier era. There have been considerable changes in the peri- and post-MI management of patients, such as administration of drugs to induce thrombolysis, early percutaneous revascularization, and treatment with aspirin and ACE inhibitors. All of these treatments alter the natural history of the post-MI patient and might influence the effects of β-blocker therapy. Furthermore, the use of β-blockers in post-MI patients with LV dysfunction or evidence of heart failure was not prospectively studied in these trials. Although LV dysfunction and/or the presence of heart failure is commonly seen as a contraindication to β-blocker therapy, post-hoc subgroup analysis of post-MI patients suggests that this approach would be ben-

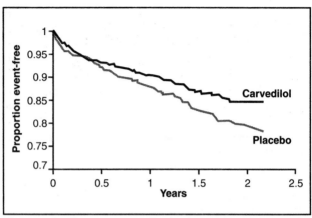

Figure 6: All-cause mortality in the CAPRICORN study. Carvedilol significantly reduced the risk of death by 23% (*P*=0.031). (Adapted from Dargie HJ: Effect of carvedilol on outcome after myocardial infarction in patients with left-ventricular dysfunction: the CAPRICORN randomised trial. *Lancet* 2001;357:1385-1390.)

eficial.[40] The Carvedilol Post-Infarct Survival Control in LV Dysfunction (CAPRICORN) trial was designed to assess the effect of a β-blocker on clinical outcomes in patients with LV dysfunction following an acute MI treated in the modern era. The study was a randomized placebo-controlled study of carvedilol compared to placebo in patients with an EF ≤0.40 with or without heart failure. Patients were included within 3 to 21 days post-MI and were receiving an ACE inhibitor at the time of randomization.

The CAPRICORN trial had co-primary end points of mortality and all-cause mortality or cardiovascular hospitalization. Whereas the combined end point showed no significant difference between the treatment groups, there was a significant 23% (*P*=0.031) reduction in all-cause mortality in the carvedilol-treated patients (Figure 6). Additionally, carvedilol therapy reduced nonfatal MI by 41%

Table 6: Dose Initiation and Target Dose of β-Blockers

Drug	Initiation Dose	Target Dose
carvedilol (Coreg®)	3.125 mg b.i.d.	25 mg b.i.d. (50 mg b.i.d. in patients >85 kg)
bisoprolol (Zebeta®)	1.25 mg q.d.	10 mg q.d.
metoprolol CR/XL (Toprol-XL®)	25 mg q.d. (12.5 mg q.d. in NYHA Class III-IV patients)	200 mg q.d.

(P=0.014), and all-cause mortality/nonfatal MI was reduced by 29% (P=0.002). These results demonstrate the efficacy of β-blockade in post-MI patients with LV dysfunction or evidence of heart failure in the modern era. They provide important information that reinforces the concept of the benefits of β-blocker therapy in a broad spectrum of patients, including the post-MI survivor with LV dysfunction. When these results were applied to this latter population, researchers anticipated that treatment of only 43 patients during the course of a year would be required to prevent one death.

How to Use β-Blockers in Heart Failure

As we have seen during the past several years, β-blockers can be safely and easily initiated, up-titrated, and maintained in most heart failure patients. The most important rule of thumb in starting a patient on a β-blocker is to start at a low dose and gradually up-titrate. Table 6 gives the starting and target doses for β-blockers that have been shown to be effective in treating heart failure patients in large-scale clinical trials. When a drug is started, patients should be counseled about the possible side effects and given instructions to weigh themselves on a daily basis (a good practice in all heart failure patients). Patients should be urged to contact the clinic if they experience increased shortness of breath, weight gain exceeding 2 pounds over any 2-day period or more than 4 pounds over the course of a 7-day period, symptoms of persistent lightheadedness, or syncope or near syncope. In the absence of these symptoms, the dose of β-blocker should be increased after (but no sooner than) 2 weeks, and the increases should continue until the target dose is reached. Whether patients require a clinic visit for each up-titration of the dose depends on the overall stability of the patient, the patient's reliability in contacting the clinic when signs of worsening heart failure occur, and the overall comfort of each prescriber in treating heart failure patients with β-blockers.

As previously noted, initiation of β-blocker therapy should be deferred in patients who are volume overloaded or acutely decompensated until they are euvolemic and their condition has stabilized. β-blockers should also be avoided in patients who have bronchospasm not related to heart failure and in patients with bradycardia. Some experts have considered the possibility of pacemaker placement in bradycardic patients in order to treat them with a β-blocker. However, there is little information in the medical literature substantiating this approach.

How to Approach Problems Related to β-Blocker Treatment of Heart Failure
Side Effects

The main side effects of β-blocker therapy of heart failure are fluid retention, hypotension, and bradycardia. A hierarchical approach to treating these side effects is outlined in Table 7.

Table 7: Management of the Most Common Side Effects of β-Blocker Therapy in Heart Failure Patients

Side Effect(s)	Strategy
Lightheadedness, hypotension	• Instruct patient to take β-blocker and ACE inhibitor (or other vasodilator) at separate times (usually 2 h apart) • If on carvedilol, take drug with meals to slow absorption • Reduce or discontinue non-ACE inhibitor vasodilators • Reduce diuretic dose in euvolemic, stable patients • Reduce ACE inhibitor dose (temporarily)
Worsening congestive signs/symptoms (eg, increased SOB, orthopnea, PND, ankle swelling)	• Assess patient's compliance with diet/drug therapy and determine if other conditions known to worsen heart failure are present • Increase diuretics • Decrease β-blocker dose if above strategies are not successful
Bradycardia	• Decrease digoxin dose (or calcium-channel blocker) • Reduce β-blocker dose • Consider pacemaker

ACE = angiotensin-converting enzyme
SOB = shortness of breath
PND = paroxysmal nocturnal dyspnea

Patients Receiving β-Blockers Who Deteriorate While on Therapy

Results from clinical trials have shown that deterioration of cardiac function caused by adding a β-blocker to the medical regimen is much less common than expected. This is related to selection (avoiding patients who are volume overloaded or decompensated) and careful dosing of the drug. When evidence of deterioration is seen, it most often occurs during initiation or up-titration of the drug. If this is the case and the patient does not respond to an increase in the diuretic dose, it is prudent to reduce (at least temporarily) the dose of the β-blocker. Although β-blocker therapy results in substantial improvement in cardiac function, relief of symptoms, and a reduction in hospitalization and emergency department visits, most patients continue to have evidence of LV dysfunction and remain at risk for deterioration. The same well-recognized factors that lead to decompensation of heart failure in patients not on β-blockers are the most common causes of clinical deterioration in patients who are receiving these agents. Thus, consideration should be given to the possibility that clinical decompensation was caused by noncompliance with the medical regimen or diet or by infection, anemia, worsening or comorbid conditions, or other causes. In cases where another cause for clinical deterioration is identified, the condition should be treated and the patient should be maintained on the β-blocker if possible. In such patients, all attempts should be made to continue β-blocker therapy.

Patients Presenting With Profound Decompensation of Heart Failure

Patients who develop profound decompensation of heart failure present a difficult problem, particularly if they require inotropic therapy to stabilize their condition. Although a direct-acting β-agonist, such as dobutamine, may work in such cases, the competition between β-blocker and β-agonist at the level of the cardiac β-receptors tends to make this approach more difficult, and higher doses of the β-agonist than might ordinarily be required are needed. A better approach is to use an agent, such as milrinone, that acts distal to the β-receptor in the adrenergic signaling pathway in stimulating myocardial contractility. In these cases, the β-blocker is continued (or sometimes reduced temporarily until the patient recovers) unless the patient is so profoundly ill that it is essential to provide as much inotropic support as possible. In these instances, β-blockers should be reduced in dose or discontinued.

Patients Who Greatly Improve (or Normalize) Their Ejection Fraction

Improvement in EF with β-blockers is common, and the usual increase is 5 to 10 EF units or more; normalization of EF may even occur in some patients. There is little reported evidence about the effects of discontinuing β-blockers in this group. When discontinuation was attempted in a small group of 24 patients who improved considerably with β-blockers, evidence of deterioration was documented in two thirds of the group.[41] Additionally, most experts are reluctant to discontinue β-blockers based on their experience that long-term neurohormonal blockade may be essential to prevent future deterioration from occurring. When the problem is explained to patients in this way, most are willing to continue β-blocker therapy indefinitely rather than risk recurrence of heart failure at some future time.

References

1.   Consensus recommendations for the management of chronic heart failure. On behalf of the membership of the advisory council to improve outcomes nationwide in heart failure. *Am J Cardiol* 1999;83:1A-38A.

2.   Eichhorn EJ, Bristow MR: Medical therapy can improve the biological properties of the chronically failing heart. A new treatment era of heart failure. *Circulation* 1996;94:2285-2296.

3.   Katz AM. In: Hosenpud JD, Greenberg BH: *Congestive Heart Failure*, 2nd ed. Philadelphia, Lippincott, Williams and Wilkins, 2000, pp 3-8.

4.   Bristow MR, Ginsburg R, Umans V, et al: β_1 and β_2-adrenergic subpopulations in nonfailing and failing human ventricular myocardium: coupling of both receptor subtypes to muscle contraction and selective β_1-receptor down regulation in heart failure. *Circ Res* 1989;59:297-309.

5.   Mann DL, Kent RL, Parsons B, et al: Adrenergic effects on the biology of the adult mammalian cardiocyte. *Circulation* 1992;85:790-804.

6.   Sutton MG, Sharpe N: Left ventricular remodeling after myocardial infarction: pathophysiology and therapy. *Circulation* 2000;101:2981-2988.

7.   Benedict CR, Weiner DH, Johnstone DE, et al: Comparative neurohormonal responses in patients with preserved and impaired left ventricular ejection fraction: results of the Studies of Left Ventricular Dysfunction (SOLVD) Registry. The SOLVD Investigators. *J Am Coll Cardiol* 1993;22:146A-153A.

8.   Francis GS, McDonald KM, Cohn JN: Neurohormonal activation in preclinical heart failure: remodeling and the potential for intervention. *Circulation* 1993;87:IV90-IV96.

9.   Cohn JN, Levine B, Olivari MT, et al: Plasma norepinephrine as a guide to prognosis in patients with chronic congestive heart failure. *N Engl J Med* 1984;311:819-823.

10.   Francis GS, Cohn JN, Johnson G, et al: Plasma norepinephrine, plasma renin activity, and congestive heart failure. Relations to survival and the effects of therapy in V-HeFT II. The V-HeFT VA Cooperative Studies Group. *Circulation* 1993;87:IV40-IV48.

11.   Waagstein F, Hjalmarson A, Varnauskas E, et al: Effect of chronic β-adrenergic receptor blockades in congestive cardiomyopathy. *Br Heart J* 1975;37:1022-1036.

12.   Swedberg K, Hjalmarson A, Waagstein F, et al: Prolongation of survival in congestive cardiomyopathy by β-receptor blockade. *Lancet* 1979;1:1374-1376.

13.   Chadda K, Goldstein S, Byington R, et al: Effect of propranolol after acute myocardial infarction in patients with congestive heart failure. *Circulation* 1986;73:503-510.

14.   Heilbrunn SM, Shah P, Bristow MR, et al: Increased β-receptor density and improved hemodynamic response to catecholamine stimulation during long-term metoprolol therapy in heart failure from dilated cardiomyopathy. *Circulation* 1989;79:483-489.

15. Eichhorn EJ, Bedotto JB, Malloy CR, et al: Effect of β-adrenergic blockade on myocardial function and energetics in congestive heart failure. Improvements in hemodynamic, contractile, and diastolic performance with bucindolol. *Circulation* 1990;82:473-483.

16. Fisher ML, Gottlieb SS, Plotnick GD, et al: Beneficial effects of metoprolol in heart failure associated with coronary artery disease: a randomized trial. *J Am Coll Cardiol* 1994;23:943-950.

17. Eichhorn EJ, Heesch CM, Barnett JH, et al: Effect of metoprolol on myocardial function and energetics in patients with nonischemic dilated cardiomyopathy: a randomized, double-blind, placebo-controlled study. *J Am Coll Cardiol* 1994;24:1310-1320.

18. Hall SA, Cigarroa CG, Marcoux L, et al: Time course of improvement in left ventricular function, mass and geometry in patients with congestive heart failure treated with β-adrenergic blockade. *J Am Coll Cardiol* 1995;25:1154-1161.

19. Olsen SL, Gilbert EM, Renlund DG, et al: Carvedilol improves left ventricular function and symptoms in chronic heart failure: a double-blind randomized study. *J Am Coll Cardiol* 1995;25:1225-1231.

20. Kaye DM, Lefkovits J, Jennings GL, et al: Adverse consequences of high sympathetic nervous activity in the failing human heart. *J Am Coll Cardiol* 1995;26:1257-1263.

21. Packer M, Carver JR, Rodeheffer RJ, et al: Effect of oral milrinone on mortality in severe chronic heart failure. The PROMISE Study Research Group. *N Engl J Med* 1991;325:1468-1475.

22. Cohn JN, Goldstein SO, Greenberg BH, et al: A dose-dependent increase in mortality with vesnarinone among patients with severe heart failure. Vesnarinone Trial Investigators. *N Engl J Med* 1998;339:1810-1816.

23. Xamoterol in severe heart failure. The Xamoterol in Severe Heart Failure Study Group. *Lancet* 1990;336:1-6.

24. Waagstein F, Bristow MR, Swedburg K, et al: Beneficial effects of metoprolol in idiopathic dilated cardiomyopathy. *Lancet* 1993;342:1441-1446.

25. A randomized trial of β-blockade in heart failure. The cardiac insufficiency bisoprolol study (CIBIS). CIBIS Investigators and Committee. *Circulation* 1994;90:1765-1773.

26. Effects of enalapril on mortality in severe congestive heart failure. Results of the Cooperative North Scandinavian Enalapril

Survival Study (CONSENSUS). The CONSENSUS Trial Study Group. *N Engl J Med* 1987;316:1429-1435.

27.   Effect of enalapril on survival in patients with reduced left ventricular ejection fractions and congestive heart failure. The SOLVD Investigators. *N Engl J Med* 1991;325:293-302.

28.   Effect on enalapril on mortality and the development of heart failure in asymptomatic patients with reduced left ventricular ejection fractions. The SOLVD Investigators. *N Engl J Med* 1992; 327:685-691.

29.   Cohn JN, Johnson G, Ziesche S, et al: A comparison of enalapril with hydralazine-isosorbide dinitrate in the treatment of chronic congestive heart failure. *N Engl J Med* 1991;325:303-310.

30.   Packer M, Bristow MR, Cohn JN, et al: The effect of carvedilol on morbidity and mortality in patients with chronic heart failure. US Carvedilol Heart Failure Study Group. *N Engl J Med* 1996; 334:1349-1355.

31.   The Cardiac Insufficiency Bisoprolol Study II (CIBIS-II): a randomized trial. *Lancet* 1999;353:9-13.

32.   Effect of metoprolol CR/XL in chronic heart failure. Metoprolol CR/XL Randomized Intervention Trial in Congestive Heart Failure (MERIT-HF). *Lancet* 1999;353:2001-2007.

33.   A trial of the β-blocker bucindolol in patients with advanced chronic heart failure. *N Engl J Med* 2001;344:1659-1667.

34.   Packer M, Coats AJ, Fowler MB, et al: Effect of carvedilol on survival in severe chronic heart failure. *N Engl J Med* 2001; 344:1651-1658.

35.   Bristow MR, Gilbert EM, Abraham WT, et al: Carvedilol produces dose-related improvements in left ventricular function and survival in subjects with chronic heart failure. MOCHA Investigators. *Circulation* 1996;94:2807-2816.

36.   Talwar KK, Bhargava B, Upasani PT, et al: Hemodynamic prediction of early intolerance and long-term effects of propranolol in dilated cardiomyopathy. *J Card Fail* 1996;2:273-277.

37.   Haber HL, Simek CL, Gimple LW, et al: Why do patients with congestive heart failure tolerate the initiation of β-blocker therapy? *Circulation* 1993;88:1610-1619.

38.   Heart Failure Society of America (HFSA) practice guidelines. HFSA guidelines for management of patients with heart failure

caused by left ventricular systolic dysfunction-pharmacological approaches. *J Card Fail* 1999;5:357-382.

39. Randomised, placebo-controlled trial of carvedilol in patients with congestive heart failure due to ischaemic heart disease. Australia/New Zealand Heart Failure Research Collaborative Group. *Lancet* 1997;349:375-380.

40. Houghton T, Freemantle N, Cleland JG: Are β-blockers effective in patients who develop heart failure soon after myocardial infarction? A meta-regression analysis of randomized trials. *Eur J Heart Fail* 2000;2:333-340.

41. Waagstein F, Caidahl K, Wallentin I, et al: Long-term β-blockade in dilated cardiomyopathy. Effects of short- and long-term metoprolol treatment followed by withdrawal and readministration of metoprolol. *Circulation* 1989;80:551-563.

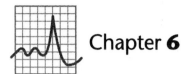

Chapter 6

Nonpharmacologic Management of Chronic Heart Failure

P harmacologic therapy for chronic heart failure with systolic left ventricular (LV) dysfunction includes ACE inhibitors, digoxin, β-blockers, diuretics, and perhaps, spironolactone (Aldactone®). With the exception of diuretics, each of these agents antagonize maladaptive neurohormonal signaling that would otherwise perpetuate LV remodeling and progressive dysfunction. The success of pharmacologic therapy can be substantially enhanced by encouraging the participation of patients and their families in complementary nonpharmacologic management strategies, including diet and nutrition, healthcare maintenance, and psychosocial or lifestyle changes. Effective disease management programs for heart failure typically encompass each of these strategies, with an emphasis on patient education, compliance, motivation, and communication. Patients who remain intolerant or moderately symptomatic after initiation of pharmacologic therapy and those with unexplained or frequent heart failure exacerbation may benefit from formal evaluation at a heart failure center or monitoring in a disease management program.

Diet and Nutrition
Sodium Restriction

In LV dysfunction, intense activation of the renin-angiotensin-aldosterone (RAA) system and the sympathetic nervous system (SNS) results in enhanced renal sodium and water retention. This activation occurs whether the abnormality is in LV filling (ie, diastolic dysfunction) or LV contractility (ie, systolic dysfunction). Pharmacologic therapy for congestive symptoms and fluid retention typically includes loop diuretics. However, while facilitating the excretion of sodium, chloride, and water, loop diuretics often induce significant potassium and magnesium wasting, with retention of organic acids, such as uric acid and nitrogenous waste products (urea).

Dietary sodium intake is an easily modifiable factor that complements pharmacologic therapy for heart failure. Sodium restriction may result in a reduction of the diuretic dose required for maintenance of both the euvolemic state and clinical stability. Salt-sensitive hypertension demonstrates the salutary relationship between higher dietary sodium intake and increasing vascular reactivity. Increasing the peripheral vascular resistance to ventricular ejection (afterload) in cardiomyopathy can result in reduced cardiac output and elevated ventricular filling pressure. Therefore, a patient with heart failure can manifest congestive symptoms whenever an acute or significant intravascular volume expansion has occurred after a 'salt challenge.'

The average daily American diet contains 8,000 to 10,000 mg sodium; certain ethnic diets are higher. A low-sodium or no-added-salt diet, as defined by the American Heart Association, is 3,000 to 4,000 mg of sodium a day. Most patients with heart failure (preserved or depressed LV function) should be advised to follow a daily dietary sodium intake between 2,000 and 3,000 mg. Further restriction to between 1,000 and 2,000 mg daily may be necessary in advanced disease with refractory fluid retention.

These recommendations arise from the clinical practice patterns of heart failure specialists, but there are no prospective data about the efficacy of isolated sodium restriction in heart failure management.

Fluid Restriction

Fluid restriction is a useful adjunct to pharmacologic therapy during hospitalization for acute heart failure exacerbation, although continuance of outpatient fluid restriction is generally reserved for advanced heart failure. For most patients, monitoring daily intake/output balance at home is cumbersome and unpleasant. Routine measurement of daily morning weight serves to monitor for either rapid or cumulative changes in weight that reflect fluid retention or loss. Most patients can be instructed to contact their health-care provider if a specified change in weight occurs, while others will benefit from the use of a diuretic 'sliding scale' or from instructions for PRN use. Restriction of daily fluid intake to between 1 and 2 L may be considered for heart failure patients with excessive oral fluid intake or with fluid retention that is not easily controlled with diuretics.

Despite these measures, patients may require escalating doses of diuretics over time. Apparent diuretic refractoriness most likely reflects unintentional or willful noncompliance with dietary recommendations and/or pharmacologic therapy. Physiologic diuretic refractoriness can also be observed with chronic loop diuretic administration primarily related to distal renal tubular hypertrophy and enhanced sodium reabsorption. Once these factors are excluded, an evaluation should be considered for untreated risk factors for disease exacerbation or underlying disease progression.

Comorbid Disease

Arteriosclerosis, hyperlipidemia, diabetes, renal insufficiency, and obesity are common comorbidities in heart failure populations. Patients and practitioners tend to underestimate the influence of these conditions on the long-term clinical course of heart failure, especially when the latter diagnosis has been classified as life-threatening. The goal of identifying medical comorbidities is to reduce risk factors for ongoing myocardial and peripheral vascular injury and, therefore, heart failure progression or decompensation. Thus, patients with hyperlipidemia or known underlying coronary or peripheral arteriosclerosis should be given specific instructions about dietary fat and cholesterol restriction. Diabetics with heart failure require aggressive management of hyperglycemia, thereby reducing both another stimulus for water retention and the long-term risk of additional end-organ damage. Patients with heart failure and significant underlying renal insufficiency (who may require protein, potassium, and other dietary constraints for preservation of electrolyte and acid-base homeostasis) are likely to benefit from formal dietary counseling. Patient (and family) counseling and education will enhance understanding and compliance for all patients as the complexity of dietary modification increases.

Weight Management

Obesity is an increasingly prevalent metabolic disorder affecting at least one third of the US population. Although the definition of obesity is controversial, the body mass index (BMI, weight divided by height [kg/m^2]) is widely used (Table 1). Obesity is independently associated with heart failure and contributes to the development of additional heart failure risk factors, including hypertension, LV hypertrophy, and diastolic filling abnormalities. Obesity is also linked to insulin resistance and glucose intolerance, hyperaldosteronism, salt sensitivity, and plasma volume expansion, creating both pressure and volume overload stress on the heart in association with increased systemic vascular resistance. The metabolic demand of excessive adipose tissue increases cardiac output requirements more than does lean body tissue at an equivalent BMI.

Cardiomyopathy with heart failure is the leading cause of death in severe obesity (Table 2). Arrhythmia risk is

Table 1: Body Mass Index Calculation for Adults > 35 Years of Age

Formulas for BMI Calculation

Weight (kg)/height squared (m^2)

or

Weight (lb) x 703/height squared (in^2)

*BMI Categories**

Underweight = < 20.7	Overweight = 27.8–31.0
Recommended weight = 20.7–27.7	Obese = ≥31

*National Center for Health Statistics standards

also increased in association with prolongation of the Q-T interval, frequently seen in morbidly obese patients. The Pickwickian syndrome (obesity-hypoventilation syndrome) is linked to pulmonary hypertension, right ventricular failure, and hypoxemia. For obesity-cardiomyopathy and obesity-hypoventilation syndrome, weight loss is an effective way to improve both symptoms and prognosis.

Therefore, in persons at risk for heart failure (Stage A; see Table 2, Chapter 2) or with diagnosed heart failure of any etiology, excessive weight represents a target for intervention. For otherwise healthy persons with a BMI of 25 to 30, the American Heart Association recommends dietary restriction and lifestyle modification. However, the defined risks of extreme caloric and carbohydrate restriction may be of particular concern for patients with heart failure, including electrolyte abnormalities and ketosis, which require frequent monitoring and physician oversight. For patients with a BMI >30, anorexigenic or antiobesity drug prescription may be considered with careful supervision, but this option must be used with caution. Fenfluramine and dexfenfluramine, now withdrawn from the market, were linked to pulmonary hypertension and valvular heart disease. For a BMI >35, gastrointestinal surgery becomes a serious option—risk for surgery depends on heart failure etiology (ie, ischemic), clinical symptoms, and hemodynamic stability. Surgical intervention is the only weight-loss therapy with reasonable long-term result maintenance.

On the opposite end of the spectrum, cardiac cachexia is a well-described phenomenon associated with intense cytokine activation (tumor necrosis factor-α [TNF-α]) and chronically low cardiac output states. Similar muscle wasting syndromes are observed in terminal cancer, acquired immune deficiency syndrome (AIDS), and chronic inflammatory disease states. In end-stage heart failure patients, however, the driving force is not an increase in tissue metabolic demand but, rather, insufficient cardiac output to meet basal tissue metabolic demands. Right-sided congestion often contributes by affecting absorption of nutrients across the gut wall. In chronic heart failure, a low BMI (underweight) is a negative prognostic marker. These patients are at extremely high risk for short-term morbidity and mortality. Treatment should be aimed at improving both the underlying cardiac condition (cardiac output) and the factors that contribute to low nutrient intake, such as depression.

Malnourished patients may benefit from referral to a nutritionist or dietitian for an optimal diet to help reverse tissue catabolism. The suggested recommended daily allowance of protein for older adults to maintain skeletal muscle health is >1 g/kg body weight. At least 40% of elderly Americans fail to meet this requirement. Some debate exists about the risk of osteoporosis caused by enhanced calciuria with higher protein intake by the elderly. It seems that a concomitant increase in fruit and/or vegetable consumption or substitution of soy or other vegetable protein for animal protein minimizes this risk. Liquid daily supplements (canned or boxed) are avail-

Table 2: BMI and Body Weight Associated With 20% and 50% Increases in Mortality From All Causes and Mortality From Cardiovascular Disease

	20% Increase			
	All-cause mortality		CVD mortality	
Group	BMI*	Weight (lb)**	BMI	Weight (lb)**
70-inch Men				
30-44 y	23.8	166	22.9	160
45-54 y	24.2	169	23.2	162
55-64 y	24.7	172	23.9	167
65-74 y	28.2	197	26.5	185
75-84 y	30.5	213	28.1	196
64-inch Women				
30-44 y	26.0	152	23.5	137
45-54 y	24.8	145	23.2	135
55-64 y	25.9	151	25.2	147
65-74 y	29.9	174	29.0	169

* A BMI of 21.0 was used as the reference value.

** For men, a height of 70 in (178 cm) and a weight of 146.5 lb (67 kg) were used as the reference values. For women, a height of 64 in (163 cm) and a weight of 122.5 lb (56 kg) were used as the reference values. These values correspond to a BMI of 21.0. Values

From Stevens J, Cai J, Pamuk ER, et al: The effect of age on the association between body-mass index and mortality. *N Engl J Med* 1998;338:1-7.

50% Increase

All-cause mortality		CVD mortality	
BMI*	Weight (lb)**	BMI*	Weight (lb)**
27.2	189	25.3	177
28.1	196	26.0	181
29.1	203	27.5	192
37.0	258	33.2	232
42.1	294	36.7	256
32.1	187	26.5	155
29.4	171	25.8	151
32.0	187	30.3	177
40.8	238	38.7	226

were not estimated for men and women ≥85 years of age and women 75 to 84 years of age, since the slopes were either negative or so small that the calculated BMI associated with a 20% increase in risk was outside the physiologic range.

BMI = body mass index
CVD = cardiovascular disease

able with variable concentrations of easily digestible protein, carbohydrates, fat, and vitamins. Many heart failure specialists suggest small, frequent meals that include these products. No data support the use of anabolic steroids or growth hormone supplementation in patients with cardiac cachexia.

Dietary Supplementation

Generally, most patients with heart failure are advised to follow a prudent diet that provides adequate protein, carbohydrates, and calories according to age, gender, and activity level. Supplementation with a daily multivitamin/mineral combination should be strongly considered, since most adult-American diets are inadequate in basic nutrient requirements. Early satiety, altered digestive efficiency from decreased absorption (gut edema), and enhanced water-soluble vitamin (particularly B vitamins) and mineral loss through diuretic administration can rapidly produce nutritional imbalance. No trials have demonstrated a survival benefit from specific supplementation of large doses of individual vitamins.

Surveys reveal that at least 50% of chronic heart failure patients consume herbal, megavitamin, or other dietary supplements to treat or prevent additional disease. When taken in this fashion, these supplements have been classified as nutraceuticals or naturoceuticals. At least 40 products now claim to have primary or secondary prevention benefits for cardiovascular conditions. The safety and efficacy of these products are not well documented. In particular, combining herbal preparations with prescription medications is not advised in the elderly or in patients with impaired physiology and metabolism.

Some specific agents should be avoided in heart failure patients because of potentially harmful actions or drug interactions. Natural or synthetic products containing ephedra (ma huang), ephedrine metabolites, or imported Chinese herbs are contraindicated in heart failure patients and have been associated with reported deaths.

184

Table 3: Summary of Dietary and Nutritional Interventions

- Sodium restriction 2,000 to 3,000 mg daily
- Fluid restriction
- Daily home weight monitoring
- Diabetes control (hyperglycemia)
- Substance abuse discontinuation
- Lipid management
- Weight loss program in severe obesity
- Nutritional supplementation

These products are marketed for reported beneficial effects such as weight loss, energy enhancement, and mental clarity. Hawthorn (*Crataegus*) products may potentiate the action of vasodilator medications and increase serum digoxin levels in vivo. Hawthorn extracts appear to have at least mild inodilator activity in vitro. Prospective, placebo-controlled, randomized trials evaluating the safety and efficacy of hawthorn in heart failure (Study of Patients Intolerant of Converting Enzyme Inhibitors [SPICE], Herbal Treatment for Patients with Congestive Heart Failure [HERB-CHF]) are under way. Many other naturoceutical products, including garlic, gingko biloba, ginseng, coenzyme Q-10, and others, have demonstrated or theoretical antiplatelet activity and/or anticoagulant interactions. Table 3 is a summary of dietary and nutritional interventions in heart failure patients.

Health-Care Maintenance

Heart failure patients should continue age- and gender-specific health screening evaluations for both primary and secondary prophylaxis against additional illness. Patients receiving frequent care from a specialist for their

Table 4: Specific Health-Care Maintenance Topics in Heart Failure Patients

- Annual influenza vaccine (Pneumovax®)
- Dental prophylaxis if appropriate
- Pain control, medication (ie, NSAID) avoidance
- Substance abuse cessation
- Sleep-disordered breathing screen
- Exercise prescription
- Routine health-care maintenance

heart condition may defer general health-care maintenance appointments with primary care providers. Specific common ailments and conditions should be reviewed and addressed with heart failure patients who have multiple care providers. A summary of relevant health-care maintenance issues can be found in Table 4.

Infection Prophylaxis

Pulmonary congestion and pulmonary hypertension each increase the risk of lung infection. Therefore, administration of pneumococcal vaccine (Pneumovax®) and annual influenza vaccines is highly recommended in heart failure patients, as is counseling patients to seek early evaluation for potentially serious infections. Over-the-counter (OTC) antihistamines, analgesics, and decongestant preparations commonly used for symptomatic relief of upper respiratory tract infections have an associated increased risk of cardiovascular side effects. Generally, most persons with heart failure may use these preparations safely for a short duration (days).

Dental and other procedural prophylaxis for bacterial endocarditis should follow standard guidelines for valvular heart disease when applicable. However, most cases of endocarditis are unrelated to invasive procedures. Maintenance of gingival health and dental hygiene is advisable. Whether functional mitral regurgitation resulting from LV chamber and valve ring dilation represents the same risk as a primary valvular disorder is unclear from available data, although most experts recommend treatment. Implanted intravascular devices, such as pacemakers or automated internal cardiac defibrillators, do not require dental prophylaxis, although many practitioners would order it shortly after implantation.

Pain Management

Some 40% to 50% of heart failure patients need analgesic medication for musculoskeletal complaints each week. Unsuspected use of nonsteroidal anti-inflammatory drugs (NSAIDs), whether prescribed or OTC, may explain worsening renal function, hyperkalemia, or increased bleeding complications among heart failure patients. NSAID use has been implicated in the onset of heart failure symptoms in the elderly, perhaps unmasking underlying ventricular dysfunction. Patients should be advised to avoid routine or long-term use of NSAIDs without careful follow-up and laboratory assessment of renal function. The risk of renal, gastrointestinal, or hematologic complications further increases with advancing age and comorbidity and in patients with reduced glomerular filtration caused by intrinsic or functional renal disease. COX-2 inhibitors may also promote fluid retention in heart failure patients. Close monitoring for unexpected weight gain after the institution of any new medication is prudent.

One particularly troublesome inflammatory condition in heart failure patients is gout. The risk of gout rises in heart failure patients with the use of diuretic medications, with an even higher risk of development seen in the obese, those with underlying renal insufficiency, and alcohol consumers. For acute gouty attacks, judicious and early colchicine administration (Colsalide®, ColBenemid®) may suffice. Intravenous administration of adrenocorticotrophic

187

hormone or hydrocortisone (40 to 80 mg) or intra-articular steroid injection are measures used by heart failure specialists as a preferred treatment to NSAID administration, particularly in patients with preexisting renal insufficiency.

Anemia Evaluation

Anemia in a patient with heart failure should be evaluated for correctable etiology rather than attributed to chronic heart disease. While it is difficult to quantitate the impact of mild to moderate chronic anemia on heart failure stability, severe anemia significantly increases the risk of myocardial ischemia, as well as the peripheral demand for cardiac output in meeting tissue metabolic oxygen requirements. With a significant influence on the perceived quality of life and functional capacity in patients with renal failure or cancer, anemia can be alleviated with the use of erythropoietin (Procrit®). However, no data clearly support erythropoietin's empirical use for anemia and chronic heart failure without renal failure.

Substance Abuse

Heart failure patients who abuse tobacco, alcohol, or illegal drugs should be repeatedly counseled to stop, although long-term abstinence rates remain disappointingly low. Nicotine has vasoconstrictor activity, which can worsen hemodynamics and antagonize vasodilator therapeutic intent. Transdermal nicotine preparations do not appear to significantly increase cardiovascular adverse events, even in high-risk patients, although physician-monitored use is advisable. Additional pharmacologic aids for tobacco withdrawal, such as bupropion (Wellbutrin®), have not been associated with increased risk of heart failure exacerbation and can be recommended for patients having difficulty with smoking cessation.

Alcohol-induced cardiomyopathy reflects toxin-induced LV dysfunction and is generally attributed to the chronic consumption of alcohol over many years. Confounding nutritional and vitamin deficiencies that coexist in chronic alcoholism may also harm ventricular function.

Renal magnesium and potassium wasting are also enhanced by ethanol. The potential for improvement or normalization of ventricular systolic function with cessation of alcohol ingestion is well recognized and correlates with improved prognosis. Whether ethanol ingestion by heart failure patients in small amounts on an infrequent basis is beneficial (vasodilatory) or harmful (toxic) is unclear; the impact on hepatic function, medication metabolism, and the tolerability of vasodilator effects must be considered in each patient.

Sleep-Disordered Breathing

Patients often ask about the use of supplemental oxygen either at night or during daily exertion; it is often used as a therapeutic adjunct in hospitalized patients during an acute exacerbation. With the exception of end-stage or refractory heart failure, oxygen supplementation is generally not indicated for chronic heart failure patients. Patients with residual resting hypoxemia after diuresis or those with exertional arterial oxygen desaturation should be evaluated for concomitant pulmonary disease, pulmonary hypertension, chronic pulmonary thromboembolic disease, silent myocardial ischemia, obesity-hypoventilation syndrome, and/or sleep-disordered breathing. Sleep-disordered breathing is prevalent in heart failure populations; formal sleep evaluation should be considered for patients who remain symptomatic after optimization of heart failure therapy. Sleep testing should also be considered for those with a positive screening questionnaire and for those whose sleep partners describe signs suggesting apnea or periodic breathing.

Insomnia is another common complaint of patients with heart failure. Chronic insomnia is associated with a risk of psychological instability and impaired daily cognitive function. After metabolic, physiologic, pharmacologic, and dietary causes are excluded, screening for urologic abnormality, sleep-disordered breathing, restless leg syndrome, depression, and anxiety disorders should be considered. Nocturnal anxiety may be a manifestation of paroxysmal nocturnal dyspnea. Pharmacologic sleep aids should rarely be used for prolonged periods because of the risk of psychological and physical dependence. Sedatives can exacerbate apnea and should initially be eliminated. Paradoxical agitation from the use of antihistamine products or benzodiazepine preparations is not uncommon.

Exercise

Regular, symptom-limited exercise should be encouraged in most heart failure patients for the well-defined benefits of conditioning and endurance on the peripheral musculature and vasculature. These benefits result in improvement in overall quality of life and exercise performance. Although exercise training is safe and improves functional capacity in stable patients with chronic heart failure, the impact of long-term exercise training on disease outcome parameters, such as morbidity and mortality, has not been formally evaluated in clinical trials. An exercise prescription, including type (aerobic vs resistance), frequency, intensity, and duration, should be provided to all patients and modified as appropriate. The use of a 6-minute walk test to measure submaximal exercise capacity provides not only an indicator of prognosis, but also a rough guideline for the activity level that the patient can easily tolerate. An alternative guide is the modified Borg scale, where a patient is instructed to achieve a level of moderate perceived exertion (Table 5).

Lifestyle and Specific Activity Issues

Chronic disease states that degrade the activities of daily living, perceived quality of life, and survival have an enormous psychological impact on patients and their families. Mood or adjustment disorders are very common. Acknowledgment of these topics is important, because patients may be reluctant to discuss them otherwise.

Mood Disorders

Depression is an independent risk factor for coronary heart disease and is increasingly common in the elderly.

Table 5: Modified Borg Scale of Perceived Exertion*

Numeric Rating of Exertion	Verbal Description of Exertion
6	None
7	Very, very light
8	Very, very light
9	Very, very light
10	Very light
11	Very light
12	**Fairly light**
13	**Somewhat difficult**
14	**Somewhat difficult**
15	**Difficult**
16	Very difficult
17	Very difficult
18	Very difficult
19	Very, very difficult
20	Very, very difficult

* For heart failure patients, the goal for regular exercise is 12 to 15 minutes.

From Borg GA: Psychophysical bases of perceived exertion. *Med Sci Sports Exerc* 1982;14:377-381.

In heart failure populations, depression has an enormous impact on quality of life and functional capacity. Furthermore, depressed mood is associated with increased morbidity (hospitalizations) and mortality. A screening assessment for situational or endogenous depression should be considered for most heart failure patients. Effective pharmacologic and cognitive therapies are available—selective serotonin reuptake inhibitors (SSRIs) are generally efficacious and safe in heart failure patients. Unlike tricyclic antidepressants (TCAs), whose anticholinergic properties increase heart rate, promote orthostatic hypotension, and alter ventricular repolarization, SSRIs have a minimal effect on hemodynamics and arrhythmia risk.

Anxiety is an associated psychological disorder that may predominate over depressive symptoms. Patients with poor insight or understanding of their diagnosis, prognosis, therapeutic plan, and treatment options often have displaced anxiety and somatization. Verbal and written educational materials allow reinforcement of coping principles. Early symptom recognition and self-monitoring techniques increase patient confidence. However, isolated nocturnal or recumbent anxiety may, in fact, represent the equivalent of paroxysmal nocturnal dyspnea. Likewise, 'panic attacks' may be precipitated by paroxysmal arrhythmia.

Sexual Dysfunction

Erectile or other sexual dysfunction is common in cardiac populations and should be discussed openly with all patients, male and female. Topics should include (when relevant) safe sexual practices, birth control, hormone supplementation, and the use of sildenafil (Viagra®) or similar drugs by male patients. Generally, use of sildenafil or similar drugs is relatively safe when heart failure symptoms are compensated and when patients are not concomitantly taking nitrate medications. Many other nonpharmacologic aids exist for erectile dysfunction, impotence, and other forms of sexual dysfunction. Patients who find it difficult to initiate discussion about these issues, or who are unaware of treatment options, may be intentionally noncompliant with heart failure medications as a means of determining their influence on sexual dysfunction. Therefore, a proactive discussion may alleviate some risk of clinical instability.

Table 6: Lifestyle and Specific Activity Issues

- Mood disorders
- Sexual dysfunction
- Employment
- Travel limitations
- Advanced directives
- End-of-life care

Employment and Travel Recommendations

Employment and travel recommendations should be individualized according to the patient's cardiovascular diagnoses, overall medical condition, and clinical stability. First, medical therapy should be optimized. Exercise evaluation using maximal oxygen consumption is often useful in determining cardiovascular reserve.

Advance Directives and End-of-Life Issues

Perhaps one of the most overlooked subjects in health-care delivery is a discussion of issues related to end-of-life events and terminal care. Although advance directives or living wills are increasingly popular, physicians may be unaware of their content unless specific inquiry is made. Alternately, patients may not consider these issues unless prompted to do so. A general discussion of prognosis and expectations related to the natural course of heart failure with a clinically stable patient is preferred. A summary of lifestyle issues related to heart failure patients can be found in Table 6.

Disease Management Programs

A variety of programs are available for assistance in the management of heart failure patients, including in-home nursing evaluation, telephone advice/triage,

Table 7: Heart Failure Disease Management Specialty Programs: Potential Components and Staffing Profile

Specialist	Requirement(s)
Physician(s)	Heart failure specialist/cardiologist with emphasis on community outreach for continuing medical education and communication with referring practitioners
RN/RNP/PA	Strong clinical skills, educator, patient advocate Educates hospital staff in continuous care coordination
Pharmacist	Medication profile review/interaction screening Lipid and anticoagulation therapy monitoring
Dietitian	Education and support (ie, label reading, recipes)
Home care services	Evaluation, transitional care Occupational and physical therapy Need for durable medical equipment must be determined Infusion services if appropriate
Social services	Transportation, meals, or in-home care assistance Information on advanced directives

Specialist	Requirement(s)
Clinical psychologist	Stress, depression, and anxiety reduction
Behavior modification	Alcohol, tobacco, or substance abuse programs
Exercise physiologist	Exercise evaluation and rehabilitation
Financial counselor	Insurance coordination, preauthorization of visits, tests
Receptionist/aide	Strong communication skills
Database manager	Chart and data tracking, outcomes statistics Cost-efficacy and care-quality data summaries
Research staff	Clinical trial conduction
Transplantation	Availability
Support groups	Interactive, educational for patients and families
Hospice/ palliative care	When appropriate, in-home or institutionally based care for end-stage patients (expected survival ≤3-6 months)

PA = physician assistant
RN = registered nurse
RNP = registered nurse practitioner

Adapted with permission from Hermann DD, Greenberg BH: Refractory heart failure: beyond standard therapy. In: Sharpe N, ed. *Heart Failure Management.* London, Martin Dunitz, 2000.

Table 8: Impact of a Comprehensive Heart Failure Treatment Program on Clinical Outcome

Year	Number of Patients	Study Type
1995	282	RCT
1997	214	PCT
1997	51	PCT
1997	149	PCT
1997	187	PCT

PCT = patient-controlled trial
RCT = randomized controlled trial

telemedicine services, computer interactive case management, and clinic-based care. Specialty heart failure centers can provide a variety of multidisciplinary services (Table 7). These programs are commonly directed by physicians and managed by nurses. Disease-specific care plans and critical pathways are commonly used by insurers, hospitals, and others to optimize resource utilization, demonstrate compliance with clinical guidelines, and evaluate quality of care.

Generally, evaluation of heart failure disease management program outcomes consistently demonstrates increased compliance with the treatment regimen and im-

Duration	Reduction in Hospitalization Rate
3 months	56% HF related 44% all cause
6 months	85% HF related 35% all cause
6 months	87% HF related 84% all cause
1 year	83% HF related
1 year	53% HF related 69% all cause

Adapted with permission from Hermann DD, Greenberg BH: Refractory heart failure: beyond standard therapy. In: Sharpe N, ed. *Heart Failure Management.* London, Martin Dunitz, 2000.

proved patient functional status, symptoms, and quality of life, as well as reduced numbers of outpatient visits, emergency evaluations, and hospital admissions (Table 8).

Suggested Readings

Ackman ML, Campbell JB, Buzak KA, et al: Use of nonprescription medications by patients with congestive heart failure. *Ann Pharmacother* 1999;33:674-679.

Adamopoulos S, Coats AJ, Brunotte F, et al: Physical training improves skeletal muscle metabolism in patients with chronic heart failure. *J Am Coll Cardiol* 1993;21:1101-1106.

Alpert MA, Terry BE, Mulekar M, et al: Cardiac morphology and left ventricular function in normotensive morbidly obese patients with and without congestive heart failure, and effect of weight loss. *Am J Cardiol* 1997;80:736-740.

Besarab A, Bolton WK, Browne JK, et al. The effects of normal as compared with low hematocrit values in patients with cardiac disease who are receiving hemodialysis and epoetin. *N Engl J Med* 1998;339:584-590.

Calle EE, Thun MJ, Petrelli JM, et al: Body-mass index and mortality in a prospective cohort of U.S. adults. *N Engl J Med* 1999;341:1097-1105.

Cheitlin MD, Hutter AM Jr, Brindis RG, et al: ACC/AHA expert consensus document. Use of sildenafil (Viagra) in patients with cardiovascular disease. American College of Cardiology/American Heart Association. *J Am Coll Cardiol* 1999;33:273-282.

Chin M, Goldman L: Factors contributing to the hospitalization of patients with congestive heart failure. *Am J Public Health* 1997;87:643-648.

Coats AJ, Adamopoulos S, Radaelli A, et al: Controlled trial of physical training in chronic heart failure. Exercise performance, hemodynamics, ventilation, and autonomic function. *Circulation* 1992;85:2119-2131.

Concise guide to the management of heart failure. World Health Organization Council on Geriatric Cardiology. Task Force on Heart Failure Education. *J Card Fail* 1996;2:153-154.

Consensus recommendations for the management of chronic heart failure. On behalf of the membership of the advisory council to improve outcomes nationwide in heart failure. *Am J Cardiol* 1999;83:1A-38A.

Davos CH, Doehner W, Rauchhaus M, et al: Obesity and survival in chronic heart failure. *Circulation* 2000;102(suppl I):I-4202.

Eckel RH: Obesity and heart disease: a statement for healthcare professionals from the Nutrition Committee, American Heart Association. *Circulation* 1997;96:3248-3250.

Fonarow GC, Stevenson LW, Walden JA, et al: Impact of a comprehensive heart failure management program on hospital readmissions and functional status of patients with advanced heart failure. *J Am Coll Cardiol* 1997;30:725-732.

Fox E, Landrum-McNiff K, Zhong Z, et al: Evaluation of prognostic criteria for determining hospice eligibility in patients with advanced lung, heart, or liver disease. SUPPORT Investigators. Study to Understand Prognoses and Preferences for Outcomes and Risks of Treatments. *JAMA* 1999;282:1638-1645.

Grady KL, Dracup K, Kennedy G, et al: Team management of patients with heart failure: a statement for healthcare professionals from the Cardiovascular Nursing Council of the American Heart Association. *Circulation* 2000;102:2443-2456.

Guidelines for the evaluation and management of heart failure. Report of the American College of Cardiology/American Heart Association Task Force on Practice Guidelines (Committee on Evaluation and Management of Heart Failure). *Circulation* 1995;92:2764-2784.

Havranek EP, Ware MG, Lowes BD: Prevalence of depression in congestive heart failure. *Am J Cardiol* 1999;84:348-350, A9.

Heerdink ER, Leufkens HG, Herings RM, et al: NSAIDs associated with increased risk of congestive heart failure in elderly patients taking diuretics. *Arch Intern Med* 1998;158:1108-1112.

Hermann DD: Acute and chronic heart failure. In: DeMaria AN, ed. *Educational Review Manual in Cardiovascular Disease*. Castle Connolly Graduate Medical Publishing, LLC, Text and CD-ROM, V 2001.

Hermann DD: Is there a role for naturoceutical agents in the management of cardiovascular disease? *Am J Cardiovasc Drugs* 2002, in press.

Hermann DD: Naturoceutical agents and cardiovascular medicine: the hope, hype and the harm. *ACC Curr J Rev* 1999;8:53-57.

Hermann DD, Greenberg B: Refractory heart failure: beyond standard therapy. In: Sharpe N, ed. *Heart Failure Management*. London, Martin Dunitz, 2000, pp 199-216.

Hermann DD, Kuiper JJ, Shabetai R, et al: Herbal, megavitamin and nutritional supplement use is very common in heart failure patient populations. *J Am Coll Cardiol* 1999;33(suppl):201A.

Horan M, Barrett F, Mulqueen M, et al: The basics of heart failure management: are they being ignored? *Eur J Heart Fail* 2000;2:101-105.

Horwich TB, Fonarow GC, Hamilton MA, et al: The relationship between obesity and mortality in patients with heart failure. *J Am Coll Cardiol* 2001;38:789-795.

Howard BV, Kritchevsky D: Phytochemicals and cardiovascular disease. A statement for healthcare professionals from the American Heart Association. *Circulation* 1997;95:2591-2593.

Hunt SA, Baker DW, Chin MH, et al: ACC/AHA guidelines for the evaluation and management of chronic heart failure in the adult. A report of the American College of Cardiology/American Heart Association Task Force on Practice Guidelines (Committee to Revise the 1995 Guidelines for the Evaluation and Management of Heart Failure). *J Am Coll Cardiol* 2001;38:2101-2113. Full text available at http://www.acc.org/clinical/guidelines/failure/hf_index.htm.

Javaheri S: Effects of continuous positive airway pressure on sleep apnea and ventricular irritability in patients with heart failure. *Circulation* 2000;101:392-397.

Konstam MA, Dracup K, Baker DW, et al: Heart failure: evaluation and care of patients with left-ventricular systolic dysfunction. *Clinical Practice Guideline No. 11.* AHCPR Publication No. 94-0612. Rockville, MD, Agency for Health Care Policy and Research, Public Health Services, US Department of Health and Human Services, 1994.

Kostis JB, Rosen RC, Cosgrove NM, et al: Nonpharmacologic therapy improves functional and emotional status in congestive heart failure. *Chest* 1994;106:996-1001.

Krachman SL, D'Alonzo GE, Berger TJ, et al: Comparison of oxygen therapy with nasal continuous positive airway pressure on Cheyne-Stokes respiration during sleep in congestive heart failure. *Chest* 1999;116:1550-1557.

Krumholz HM, Phillips RS, Hamel MB, et al: Resuscitation preferences among patients with severe congestive heart failure: results from the SUPPORT project. Study to Understand Prognoses and Preferences for Outcomes and Risks of Treatments. *Circulation* 1998;98:648-655.

Mashour NH, Lin GI, Frishman WH. Herbal medicine for the treatment of cardiovascular disease: clinical considerations. *Arch Intern Med* 1998;158:2225-2234.

Massie BM, Shah NB: Evolving trends in the epidemiologic factors of heart failure: rationale for preventive strategies and comprehensive disease management. *Am Heart J* 1997;133:703-712.

McKelvie RS, Teo KK, McCartney N, et al: Effects of exercise training in patients with congestive heart failure: a critical review. *J Am Coll Cardiol* 1995;25:789-796.

Naughton MT, Bradley TD: Sleep apnea in congestive heart failure. *Clin Chest Med* 1998;19:99-113.

NHLBI Obesity Education Initiative Expert Panel: *Clinical Guidelines on Identification, Evaluation, and Treatment of Overweight and Obesity in Adults: The Evidence Report*. Bethesda, MD, National Institutes of Health, National Heart, Lung, and Blood Institute, 1998.

Philbin EF: Comprehensive multidisciplinary programs for the management of patients with congestive heart failure. *J Gen Intern Med* 1999;14:130-135.

Rich MW: Heart failure disease management: a critical review. *J Card Fail* 1999;5:64-75.

Rich MW, Beckham V, Wittenberg C, et al: A multidisciplinary intervention to prevent the readmission of elderly patients with congestive heart failure. *N Engl J Med* 1995;333:1190-1195.

Rich MW, Nease RF: Cost-effectiveness analysis in clinical practice: the case of heart failure. *Arch Intern Med* 1999;159:1690-1700.

Stevens J, Cai J, Pamuk ER, et al: The effect of age on the association between body-mass index and mortality. *N Engl J Med* 1998; 338:1-7.

Stevenson LW: Rites and responsibility for resuscitation in heart failure: tread gently on the thin places [editorial]. *Circulation* 1998;98:619-622.

Swan JW, Anker SD, Walton C, et al: Insulin resistance in chronic heart failure: relation to severity and etiology of heart failure. *J Am Coll Cardiol* 1997;30:527-532.

The care of dying patients: a position statement from the American Geriatrics Society. AGS Ethics Committee. *J Am Geriatr Soc* 1995;43:577-578.

Tkacova R, Rankin F, Fitzgerald FS, et al: Effects of continuous positive airway pressure on obstructive sleep apnea and left ventricular afterload in patients with heart failure. *Circulation* 1998;98:2269-2275.

Wenger NK, Froelicher ES, Smith LK et al: Cardiac rehabilitation as secondary prevention. *Clinical Practice Guideline No.* 17. AHCPR Publication No. 96-0672. Rockville, MD, US Department of Health and Human Services, Public Health Service, Agency for Health Care Policy and Research and the National Heart, Lung, and Blood Institute, October 1995.

Willet WC, Dietz WH, Colditz GA: Guidelines for healthy weight. *N Engl J Med* 1999;341:427-434.

Chapter 7

Management of Acute Decompensated Heart Failure

A cute decompensated heart failure (ADHF) resulting in hospitalization remains a major public health issue with a tremendous attributable cost in healthcare expenditures and lives lost. The frequency of heart failure hospitalization has risen, paralleling the increasing incidence and prevalence of heart failure in both women and men (Figure 1). This represents approximately 1 million hospital admissions annually in the United States, an increase of more than 50% over the past 10 years. Medicare data reveal that ADHF is the most common admitting diagnosis in persons older than 65 years of age, and more than 80% of patients seeking emergency care for ADHF are subsequently hospitalized. Hospital-based acute care accounts for approximately 75% of the total healthcare cost of heart failure management, approximately $15 billion annually.

Despite the enormous significance of this problem, delineation of optimal therapeutic approaches to ADHF therapy through classical clinical trials has been relatively sparse. Most approaches focus on disease identification and management protocols applied through critical path-

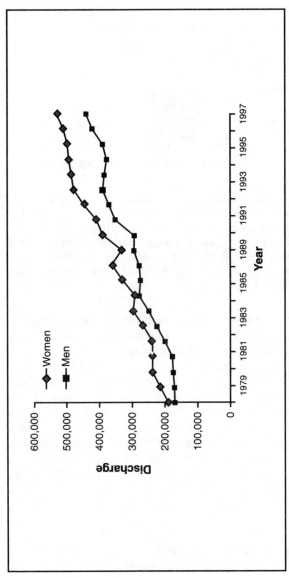

Figure 1: Heart failure hospitalization data from the 1988 Statistical Update, National Center for Health Statistics. Data includes both living and deceased discharges.

203

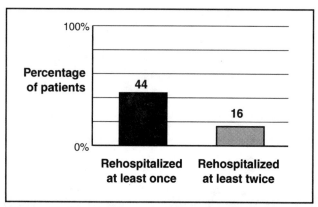

Figure 2: Six-month readmission rates for survivors of ADHF hospitalization. Data on rehospitalization frequency from 17,448 Medicare patients. Adapted from Krumholz HM, Parent EM, Tu N, et al: Readmission after hospitalization for congestive heart failure among Medicare beneficiaries. *Arch Intern Med* 1997;157:99-104.

ways for chronic heart failure therapy initiation in the hospital setting. The goal of such pathways is to optimize cost efficiency, reduce hospital length of stay and readmission rates, and improve patient survival by triggering the institution of appropriate chronic maintenance therapy. As a result, for ADHF, hospital length of stay has decreased to an average of 5 to 6 days (a 30% reduction). However, readmission rates remain unacceptably high, with 20% to 25% occurring within 30 days of hospital discharge and 50% within 6 months. Figure 2 shows the readmission rate among Medicare patient populations, where the age-adjusted prevalence of chronic heart failure is 2.3% in men and 1.5% in women. Unfortunately, posthospitalization short-term heart failure mortality rates have not significantly decreased despite tremendous advances in chronic heart failure therapy, such that hospitalization in itself carries prognostic relevance. The 30-

Table 1: Principles in the Management of ADHF

- Verify that the diagnosis of ADHF is correct by considering appropriate differential diagnoses that may mimic this clinically defined syndrome.

- If unknown, establish the etiology and extent of ventricular dysfunction and institute appropriate therapy. Is systolic ventricular function impaired (LVEF <0.40) or preserved? Is myocardial ischemia present? Is there an arrhythmia?

- Provide symptomatic improvement and achieve hemodynamic stability as the initial goals of therapy.

- Evaluate and treat reversible provocative or exacerbating conditions and comorbidities.

- Initiate long-term, stepwise therapy necessary to reduce progressive ventricular remodeling and promote clinical stability.

- Provide appropriate interval follow-up and ongoing patient education as a critical portion of the treatment plan.

LVEF = left ventricular ejection fraction

---

day mortality risk following heart failure hospitalization ranges between 5% and 10%, increasing to 20% to 40% at 6 to 12 months. The impetus for developing new pharmacologic approaches for the treatment of ADHF is, therefore, strong. The goal of emerging effective therapies is to produce a reduction in the frequency of recurrent hospitalization and improve short-term morbidity and mortality rates.

This chapter provides an overview of ADHF treatment strategies and pharmacologic options. Promising new agents

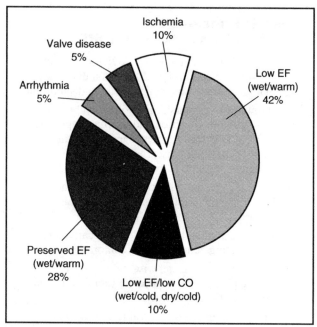

Figure 3: Estimated percentage of ADHF patients with presenting symptoms or signs. Excluding patients with acute myocardial infarction; only a small proportion of patients admitted with ADHF are in overt cardiogenic shock (wet/cold). EF=ejection fraction; CO=cardiac output. Stevenson LW, Massie BM, Francis GS, et al: Optimizing therapy for complex or refractory heart failure: a management algorithm. *Am Heart J* 1998;135:S293-S309.

now in various phases of clinical trial evaluation will also be summarized. A practical approach to hospital-based ADHF management is summarized in Table 1.

Patient Presentation

ADHF is either new-onset heart failure or significant symptomatic worsening of a previously diagnosed condi-

Table 2: Etiology of New-Onset ADHF

- Acute myocardial infarction
- Acute coronary syndromes without infarction
- Hypertensive crisis (excessive afterload)
- Acute myocarditis (rare)
- Acute valvular regurgitation (mitral or aortic)
- Sustained tachyarrhythmia
- Papillary muscle or ventricular septal rupture
- Ruptured chordae tendineae (degenerative)
- Acute secondary myocardial dysfunction (eg, sepsis, toxemia)

tion. Severe dyspnea is the predominant symptom precipitating hospitalization. Patients presenting with ADHF generally develop symptoms rapidly, within minutes to days. Approximately 80% of ADHF hospitalizations occur among patients with previously diagnosed heart failure. Figure 3 illustrates the estimated frequency of presenting signs and the nature of ventricular dysfunction in ADHF patients without acute myocardial infarction (MI). Most have abnormal systolic function when assessed acutely; patients with preserved systolic function defined as an ejection fraction >0.40 account for approximately one third of hospital admissions.

Whether the patient has a history of cardiovascular disease or ventricular dysfunction, hospitalization alone generally indicates a patient at high risk for morbidity and mortality. The patient with new-onset ADHF is much more likely to have a condition resulting from acute mechanical ventricular dysfunction, as shown in Table 2. Severe anemia, sepsis or toxemia, hypoxemia, acidosis, hypo- or hypervolemia, and many other conditions can precipitate secondary myocardial dysfunction (systolic or diastolic).

Table 3: Precipitating or Exacerbating Factors for ADHF*

- Medication noncompliance
- Silent or overt ischemia/infarction
- Dietary sodium indiscretion
- Untreated hypertension
- Inadequate medical therapy
- Acute or chronic infection
- Uncontrolled hyperglycemia
- Thyroid dysfunction
- Inadequate follow-up
- Atrial fibrillation (new or rapid)
- Other arrhythmia
- Renal or hepatic insufficiency
- Nephrosis or cirrhosis
- Pulmonary embolism or hypertension
- Substance abuse (alcohol, stimulants)
- Worsening valvular or ventricular function
- Over-the-counter drug or supplement use
- Iatrogenic factors
- Pregnancy
- Severe anemia (chronic)

*Patients with previously diagnosed chronic heart failure.

In the patient with *previously diagnosed* chronic heart failure, common reasons for acute decompensation or symptomatic exacerbation include medical or dietary non-

Table 4: Indications for Intensive Care Monitoring in ADHF

- Evidence of myocardial infarction, acute coronary syndrome, or mechanical complication

- Significant ventricular or supraventricular arrhythmia

- Compromised respiratory function (profound tachypnea, hypoxemia, or severe comorbid lung disease)

- Evidence of low cardiac output (impaired perfusion, mentation, hypotension, vasoconstriction, oliguria)

- Anticipated need for hemodynamic monitoring or frequent vital sign reassessment

- Severe comorbid disease (sepsis, ketoacidosis, preexisting renal insufficiency)

compliance (willful or inadvertent); abuse of substances such as stimulants, nicotine, sedatives, or alcohol; and inadequate outpatient therapy or follow-up. Untreated systemic or pulmonary hypertension, infection, poorly controlled diabetes, arrhythmias, and inadequate or inappropriate prescribed or self-administered medications, such as nonsteroidal anti-inflammatory drugs (NSAIDs), are also frequently observed. Seeking a correctable cause for ADHF is important, as progression of underlying disease reflecting heart failure refractory to standard therapy connotes a poor short-term prognosis. The latter warrants aggressive management strategies, such as referral to a heart failure and/or cardiac transplant program. Table 3 summarizes common factors known to increase the likelihood of clinical decompensation in chronic heart failure.

Determining the appropriate level of care depends on the assessment of patients' vital signs and examination findings, the interval frequency of monitoring procedures, the nature of planned interventions, clinical hemodynamic stability, and the initial symptomatic response to therapy. Intensive care monitoring should be strongly considered whenever there are symptoms or signs of reduced cardiac output with or without pulmonary edema. Table 4 details additional indications for intensive care unit admission for a patient with ADHF.

Physical findings of ADHF are more sensitive and specific than the same signs in chronic heart failure. Common findings include tachypnea, often with use of accessory muscles; limited inspiratory diaphragmatic excursion because of increased lung stiffness; rales; and/or wheezing. Acute pulmonary edema demonstrated on chest radiography and hypoxemia are not uncommon. However, signs of pulmonary hypertension or systemic congestion may be absent. An evaluation of cardiac output includes an assessment of mentation, peripheral pulses and perfusion, and urine output. Determining the presence, nature, and etiology of ventricular dysfunction is key to proper management. Determining whether ventricular systolic function is impaired or preserved enables directed rather than empiric therapy.

Stevenson et al suggested a management scheme for ADHF in the chronic heart failure patient with a depressed ejection fraction based on symptoms and signs of congestion and perfusion. Patients with dyspnea, edema, or other evidence of volume overload are considered *wet*; those without intravascular volume expansion or who are clinically volume depleted are considered *dry*. The next classification is based on an assessment of cardiac output and peripheral perfusion, with the patient categorized as either *warm* or *cold*. The relative frequency of predominant symptoms or signs on presentation with ADHF is shown in Figure 3.

Bedside echocardiography is a valuable tool for the evaluation of anatomic and functional abnormalities, al-

Table 5: Goals for ADHF Therapy

Acute/Immediate Management Goals

- Maintain or restore organ function and perfusion
- Symptom alleviation (pulmonary congestion relief)
- Stabilize patient for early ICU discharge

Transitional (Predischarge) Management Goals

- Eliminate residual volume overload
- Initiate effective outpatient maintenance regimen
- Shorten length of stay
- Plan for definitive therapy (surgery, device, medical)

Intermediate/Long-term Management Goals

- Prevent early deterioration and hospital recidivism
- Improve prognosis
- Restore functional capacity

though if it is not immediately available, initiation of treatment should not be delayed. Other evaluation methods, such as impedance plethysmography, can provide noninvasive estimates of cardiac output, total lung water, systemic vascular resistance, and other hemodynamic variables. Whether this adds information to the clinical history and examination in ADHF is unknown.

Medical Therapy for ADHF

Therapy for ADHF can be divided into chronologic categories for acute/immediate therapy, subacute or transitional therapy, and intermediate/long-term management. Each phase during acute hospitalization has independent goals (Table 5).

Table 6: Common Hemodynamic Patterns in the Differential Diagnosis of ADHF*

	Cardiac Output	Right Atrial Pressure
Acute (cardiac) pulmonary edema	Variable	→ or ↑
Cardiogenic shock (acute infarction)	⇓	↑
Acute decompensated heart failure (ADHF)	↓ to ⇓	↑
Acute right ventricular failure	↓	⇑

* ADHF has hemodynamic features congruent with those of acute cardiogenic shock in the setting of acute myocardial infarction. Higher pulmonary artery pressures are commonly observed when preexisting

Initial Therapy

For the emergency department patient, obtain vital signs, provide supplemental oxygen, and establish venous access. In the absence of symptomatic hypotension or pulmonary edema, placing the patient in a semirecumbent or seated position facilitates care. Obtain a 12-lead electrocardiogram (EKG) and institute telemetry monitoring if the potential

Pulmonary Artery Pressure	Pulmonary Wedge Pressure	Systemic Vascular Resistance	Mixed Venous Oxygen Saturation
↑	⇑	Variable	Variable
↑	↑	⇑	↓ to ⇓
⇑	⇑	↑	↓ to ⇓
→ to ↓	→ to ↓	↑	↑

chronic heart failure is long-standing, enabling cardiac output compensation or preservation at the expense of greatly increased filling pressures.

for ischemia, infarction, or arrhythmia is clinically suspect. Arterial blood gas analysis and/or determination of arterial oxygen saturation by pulse oximetry should be performed, especially if concomitant lung disease is present.

While obtaining a history and performing a physical assessment, obtain a chest radiograph and laboratory evaluation results, including a complete blood count

Table 7: Intravenous Agents Used in Acute and Chronic Heart Failure

Agent	Typical Dose Range	Action/Class
Nitroglycerin	10-200 μg/min	Venodilator, coronary vasodilator
Nitroprusside	0.1-5 μg/kg/min	Venodilator, arterial vasodilator
Dobutamine	3-15 μg/kg/min	+Inotrope, β-adrenergic agonist, dose-dependent $\beta_1 > \beta_2$ effects
Dopamine	2-20 μg/kg/min	+Inotrope, β-adrenergic and dopaminergic agonist, dose-dependent $\beta_1 > \beta_2$ effects
Isoproterenol	0.01-0.1 μg/kg/min	+Inotrope, β_1, β_2-adrenergic agonist, vasodilator

Indication	1° Effect	Comment
Myocardial ischemia, elevated PAWP, HTN	↓Preload ↓Mild afterload	Rapid onset
HTN crisis, elevated PAWP, acute aortic or mitral regurgitation	↓↓Afterload, ↓preload	Risk coronary steal from hypotension, thiocyanate toxicity
Insufficient cardiac output with or without congestion/hypotension	↑Cardiac output and stroke volume	Tachyphylaxis observed with prolonged use, risk tachycardia, ischemia, eosinophilia observed due to vehicle used
Insufficient cardiac output with relative hypotension, reduced renal perfusion with oliguria	Cardiac output and ↑stroke volume, ↑renal blood flow	Tachycardia, ischemia, arrhythmia risk, at high dose has α-pressor action and increases afterload
Bradycardia, insufficient cardiac output	↑Heart rate and cardiac output, ↑BP	Tachycardia, ischemia, hypotension

(continued on next page)

215

Table 7: Intravenous Agents Used in Acute and Chronic Heart Failure *(continued)*

Agent	Typical Dose Range	Action/Class
Norepinephrine	0.01-0.1 µg/kg/min	+Inotrope, β-adrenergic agonist, dose-dependent β_1, α-pressor effects = vasoconstriction
Milrinone/ amrinone	0.3-1.0 µg/kg/min/ 5-10 µg/kg/min	Inotrope and vasodilator, via phosphodiesterase inhibition
Phenylephrine	10-200 µg/min	β_1-mediated vasoconstriction
Morphine sulfate	1-5 mg	Venodilator, analgesic

(CBC) and a chemistry panel with electrolytes, magnesium, creatinine, blood urea nitrogen (BUN), glucose, and albumin. Cardiac enzymes and other laboratory studies (toxicology, coagulation studies, and thyroid panel) should be measured if clinically appropriate. A comparison of the acute hemodynamic profile typically observed in ADHF and the profiles of other conditions presenting with acute dyspnea and/or hypoperfusion is shown in Table 6.

Generally, initial treatment measures are intended to provide rapid symptom reduction or relief and hemodynamic stabilization. Diuretics are a cornerstone treatment

Indication	1° Effect	Comment
Severe hypotension despite use of another inotrope or phenylephrine	Vasoconstriction ↑↑Afterload	High-risk tachycardia, arrhythmia, ischemia. Used rarely until cause of hypotension treated.
Low cardiac output, high PCWP, pulmonary hypertension	↓Afterload and preload, ↑cardiac output	Long t-1/2, delay to peak effect if loading dose omitted. Risk arrhythmia, hypotension. Amrinone has risk of thrombocytopenia.
Hypotension, low PVR states (sepsis)	↑Afterload	Use only transiently until cause of hypotension treated.
Severe pain, high PAWP, ischemia	↓Preload	May cause hypotension, respiratory depression.

of acute congestive symptoms related to sodium or volume overload and should be administered intravenously (IV) in the acute setting to minimize onset of action. Rapid bolus administration of loop diuretics can have undesired systemic vasoconstrictor effects (see Chapter 3). Vasodilators, inotropic agents, inodilators, or vasopressor drugs may be necessary when signs of reduced cardiac output persist and should be used as indicated (Table 7). Stevenson et al devised a simple classification for treatment based on recognition of the physical signs reflecting the most acute hemodynamic change. Determining whether

Table 8: Initial Emergency Department Treatment of ADHF

Optimize oxygenation

- O_2
- BiPAP®
- CPAP
- Mechanical ventilation

Assess hemodynamics

- *'Wet':* Nitrates, diuretics, nesiritide, opiates
- *'Cold':* Inotropes, dopamine, inodilators
- *Hypotensive:* Dopamine or dobutamine
- *Hypertensive:* Nitrates, nitroprusside, IV vasodilators

Maintain organ (renal) perfusion

- *'Cold':* Inotropes, dopamine, inodilators

Reduce volume overload

- *'Wet':* Diuretics, vasodilators

Treat accompanying conditions

- Ischemia, acute coronary syndromes
- Arrhythmias
- Noncardiac comorbidities

the patient is warm (perfused) or cold (vasoconstricted) serves as a surrogate for cardiac output. Whether the patient is wet (volume overloaded or congested) or dry (not congested) correlates with left ventricular filling pressures. The patient's hemodynamic subset assists in determining the level of care needed and the most effective therapy (Table 8 and Figure 4). Deciding when to use intra-aortic

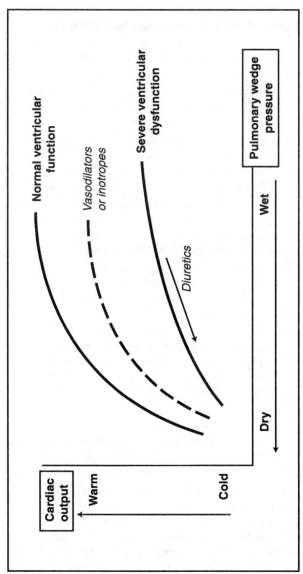

Figure 4: Drug effects on the Frank-Starling curve.

219

Table 9: ACC Consensus Indications for Right Heart Catheterization in Acute MI with ADHF

- Differentiation between cardiogenic and hypovolemic shock when initial therapy with intravascular volume expansion and low doses of inotropic drugs has failed.

- Guidance of management of cardiogenic shock with pharmacologic and/or mechanical support in patients with and without coronary reperfusion therapy.

- Short-term guidance of pharmacologic and/or mechanical management of acute mitral regurgitation (with or without disruption of the mitral valve) before surgical correction.

- Establishment of severity of left-to-right shunting and short-term guidance of pharmacologic and/or mechanical management of ventricular septal rupture before surgical correction.

- Guidance of management of right ventricular infarction with hypotension and/or signs of low cardiac output not responding to intravascular volume expansion, low doses of inotropic drugs, and/or restoration of heart rate and atrioventricular synchrony.

- Guidance of management of acute pulmonary edema not responding to treatment with diuretic drugs, nitroglycerin and other vasodilator agents, and low doses of inotropic drugs.

balloon counterpulsation or other circulatory assist devices is reviewed below.

Right heart catheterization is useful but not always necessary to initiate therapy. The American College of Cardiology (ACC) consensus agreement for when to perform this procedure in the setting of MI with evidence of heart failure can be found in Table 9. The ACC consensus agreement for when to perform this procedure in the setting of heart failure exacerbation can be found in Table 10.

Intravenous Vasodilator Therapy

The acutely decompensated heart is extremely sensitive to intrinsic loading conditions. Decreasing preload with diuretics and/or venodilators results in symptomatic relief of congestion caused by reduced ventricular filling pressure. However, in the setting of excessive systemic vascular resistance, afterload reduction accomplished through vasodilator therapy has a more substantial effect on systolic function and cardiac output. A summary of agents is reviewed in Table 7. Combinations of these agents may be used for synergy when monotherapy does not achieve the desired clinical effect.

Nitroglycerin has a rapid onset of action (3 to 5 minutes) by virtually any route of administration. Continuous IV administration allows rapid titration to hemodynamic goals or relief of symptoms of myocardial ischemia. Nitroglycerin has predominantly venodilatory effects but possesses mild arteriolar vasodilating activity. Nitroglycerin is most effective in cardiogenic pulmonary edema as a result of myocardial ischemia. Pharmacodynamic tolerance can occur in as few as 4 to 8 hours of continuous infusion therapy but can usually be overcome by a dose increase. Toxicity and rebound hemodynamic deterioration is uncommon, even with prolonged administration.

Sodium nitroprusside is an exceedingly powerful smooth-muscle vasodilator, resulting in arteriolar and venodilator activity. It should be used cautiously in the setting of acute myocardial ischemia or infarction. A reduction in the mean arterial pressure (coronary perfusion pressure) along with coronary vasodilation can produce a 'steal' phenomenon, worsening myocardial blood flow to

Table 10: ACC Consensus Indications for Right Heart Catheterization in ADHF

- Differentiation between hemodynamic and permeability pulmonary edema or dyspnea (or determination of the contribution of left heart failure to respiratory insufficiency in patients with concurrent cardiac and pulmonary disease) when a trial of diuretic and/or vasodilator therapy has failed or is associated with high risk.

- Differentiation between cardiogenic and noncardiogenic shock when a trial of intravascular volume expansion has failed or is associated with high risk; guidance of pharmacologic and/or mechanical support.

- Guidance of therapy in patients with concomitant manifestations of 'forward' (hypotension, oliguria, and/or azotemia) and 'backward' (dyspnea and/or hypoxemia) heart failure.

- Guidance of perioperative management in selected patients with decompensated heart failure undergoing intermediate or high-risk noncardiac surgery.

- Determination of whether pericardial tamponade is present when clinical assessment is inconclusive and echocardiography is unavailable, technically inadequate, or nondiagnostic. Low doses of inotropic drugs and/or restoration of heart rate and atrioventricular synchrony.

- Detection of the presence of pulmonary vasoconstriction and determination of its reversibility in patients being considered for heart transplantation.

ischemic territories. Furthermore, rapid reduction in systemic arterial pressure can stimulate a reflex tachycardia, creating an increased myocardial oxygen demand.

Nitroprusside is most useful in the setting of heart failure caused by uncontrolled 'malignant' hypertension and acute severe mitral or aortic valvular regurgitation. Long-term use (>72 hours) is not advisable because of the well-defined risk of thiocyanate and cyanide toxicity, particularly in patients with renal insufficiency. Rebound hypertension and recurrent hemodynamic deterioration have been observed with rapid discontinuation; a more gradual dose withdrawal with concomitant upward titration of oral vasodilator medications is practical.

Positive Inotropic Agents and Inodilator Therapy

Dobutamine, dopamine, and other sympathomimetics. The choice of sympathomimetic agent used in ADHF depends on the desired hemodynamic effect. Dobutamine (Dobutrex®) and dopamine are the most commonly used agents because they are most likely to augment stroke volume and cardiac output without adverse effects on mean arterial pressure or systemic vascular resistance via peripheral adrenergic receptor stimulation (Figure 5). The role of these agents in the acute management of patients with systolic heart failure exacerbation who are receiving β-blockers as part of their medical regimen is unclear.

Dobutamine and dopamine exert primarily β_1-adrenergic-receptor-mediated action with dose-dependent effects. However, the observed clinical response caused by receptor stimulation by these agents may be affected by alterations in sympathetic tone and β-receptor down-regulation in chronic heart failure. Tolerance has been observed with long-term administration. A short half-life is advantageous when unexpected hypotension, tachycardia, or tachyarrhythmia results.

Other phosphodiesterase inhibitors. Phosphodiesterase (PDE) inhibition results in an increase in intracellular cyclic adenosine monophosphate, which, in turn, augments

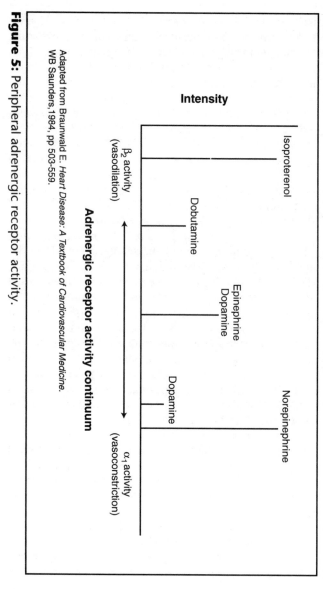

Figure 5: Peripheral adrenergic receptor activity.

Adapted from Braunwald E. *Heart Disease: A Textbook of Cardiovascular Medicine.* WB Saunders,1984, pp 503-559.

sarcolemmal calcium uptake. PDE inhibitors produce positive myocardial inotropic effects and peripheral and pulmonary vasodilation caused by smooth muscle relaxation. Generally, loading doses are considered unnecessary and tend to produce excessive hypotension. Steady-state hemodynamic actions generally include an increase in stroke volume and cardiac index with decreases in pulmonary capillary wedge pressure and systemic vascular resistance with little change in heart rate. Tolerance has not been observed, and the risk of arrhythmia is generally less than that of dobutamine because of the absence of β-receptor stimulation.

Milrinone (Primacor®) is the PDE inhibitor most widely used for the acute management of decompensated heart failure. Its anecdotal use is increasing as a 'bridge to β-blockade' for long-term management of patients with severe refractory heart failure who are unable to tolerate β-blocker therapy. Its limitations include its relatively high cost (compared to dobutamine) and concern over the risk of increased mortality with long-term administration, as has been observed in clinical trials with oral PDE inhibitors. The Prospective, Randomized Milrinone Survival Evaluation (PROMISE) trial was stopped prematurely because of significantly increased mortality in the patients randomized to oral milrinone therapy. Trials with oral enoximone and vesnarinone have also demonstrated deleterious effects on long-term survival.

The Outcomes of a Prospective Trial of Intravenous Milrinone for Exacerbations of Chronic Heart Failure (OPTIME) trial was designed with the hypothesis that in patients hospitalized for ADHF (not requiring inotropic therapy), treatment with IV milrinone as an adjunct to standard medical care during hospitalization may improve short- and intermediate-term (60-day) outcomes. The primary end point was the change in total cardiovascular hospitalization days during the 60-day period after enrollment, and secondary evaluation of total mortal-

225

Table 11: OPTIME Trial Data

	Placebo	Milrinone	P Value
Total mortality (%)			
In-hospital	2.3	3.6	0.104
Day 60	8.9	10.3	0.441
Morbidity/mortality (%)			
60-day death or heart failure rehospitalization	35.3	35.0	0.914

ity and hospitalization were planned prospectively. Eligible patients had preexisting systolic left ventricular dysfunction with symptomatic exacerbation of congestive symptoms—otherwise, their care remained under the direction of their admitting primary care physician. Patients were randomized within 48 hours of admission to receive either milrinone (0.5 µg/kg/min) or placebo infusion for an additional 48 hours. When milrinone was used in this fashion, there was no reduction in the average hospital length of stay (approximately +6/-13 days), 60-day mortality rate (2% to 3%), or the combined mortality or repeated hospitalization rate (35%). There was a significant increase in adverse events (primarily symptomatic sustained hypotension) in the patients receiving milrinone (Table 11). Although the design of the trial remains controversial, the empiric use of milrinone as prescribed in the OPTIME trial for the 'warm and wet' patient appears to have limited value.

Supportive Mechanical Assist Devices

For patients with systolic (and occasionally diastolic) ventricular dysfunction who remain hemodynamically unstable and are unresponsive to or intolerant of medical management or require extensive pharmacologic support, the use of circulatory assist devices often provides a means for hemodynamic stabilization. Before using these devices, clinicians must consider the clinical setting and whether the patient's current condition is correctable or at least partially reversible over time with supportive care (eg, myocarditis, sepsis, renal failure), revascularization (eg, ischemia, infarction), or other surgical intervention (valve repair or replacement, cardiac transplantation). Discussion of the use of these therapies is beyond the scope of this chapter.

Mechanical support is only intended to be used as a bridge to definitive therapy or recovery. Patients with severe comorbidity, such as cancer, multiorgan failure, advanced age, or anoxic brain injury following cardiac arrest, warrant frank preimplantation ethical consideration of the end points of care. Commonly used devices include the percutaneously placed intra-aortic balloon pump or hemopump, extracorporeal membrane oxygenating systems, hemofiltration, dialysis, and implanted ventricular assist devices. The options and/or choice of therapy used depend on local availability and staff experience.

New or Investigational Agents

Brain natriuretic peptide (BNP, nesiritide [Natrecor®]) is one of four endogenous natriuretic peptides originally identified in brain tissue, but primarily synthesized in ventricular myocardium. Endogenous BNP acts as both an arterial dilator and venodilator and has other beneficial actions in chronic heart failure (Table 12).

Infusion of synthetic BNP in ADHF produces dose-dependent improvement in central hemodynamics and symptoms. The Vasodilation in the Management of Acute Congestive Heart Failure (VMAC) trial had the primary objective of comparing the hemodynamic and clinical effects of a nesiritide infusion to placebo or nitroglycerin when added to standard therapy in the treatment of decompensated heart failure. The results showed that nesiritide was equally or more

Table 12: Endogenous Natriuretic Peptides

Short-term Benefits
- Vasodilation
- Reduction in left and right heart filling pressures
- Suppression of plasma norepinephrine levels
- Reduction in plasma arginine vasopressin (AVP), renin, and aldosterone activities

Long-term Benefits (Theoretical)
- Inhibition of vascular smooth muscle
- Inhibition of myocyte hypertrophy
- Inhibition of interstitial fibrosis

effective in ADHF than nitroglycerin or placebo, decreasing pulmonary capillary wedge pressure further and more rapidly while reducing systemic vascular resistance and increasing cardiac output without inotropic stimulation (Figure 6). In the VMAC trial, no difference was observed in the 30-day readmission rate for the groups receiving nitroglycerin or nesiritide (20% to 23%). However, when compared with IV dobutamine administration in another study, readmissions were significantly reduced with nesiritide (Figure 7).

Nesiritide is less potent and less toxic than nitroprusside, although symptomatic hypotension is the major limiting side effect. Frequency of side effects, which varied significantly from placebo in dose-finding and efficacy trials with nesiritide, is shown in Table 13. In patients with chronic heart failure, nesiritide has only mild intrinsic diuretic and natriuretic activity.

Recently, the Food and Drug Administration (FDA) approved using nesiritide as a vasodilator agent in acute decompensated congestive heart failure, based on its superior-

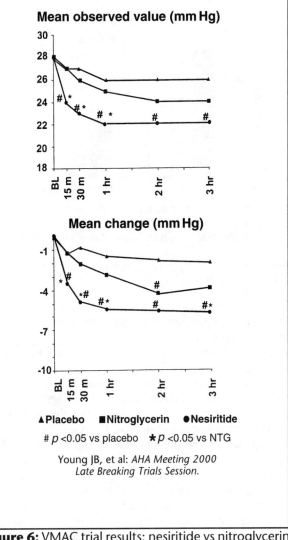

Figure 6: VMAC trial results: nesiritide vs nitroglycerin and placebo.

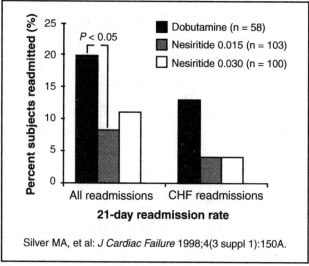

Silver MA, et al: *J Cardiac Failure* 1998;4(3 suppl 1):150A.

Figure 7: Hospital readmission rates comparing nesiritide to dobutamine.

ity in producing symptomatic relief reflecting clinical improvement (global clinical status) at 6 hours (Figure 8). A suggested treatment algorithm for when and how to use nesiritide is shown in Figure 9.

Calcium-sensitizing agents are being evaluated in clinical trials for use in ADHF. Most of these agents differ in mechanism from the drugs available now that increase intracellular calcium concentration. Calcium entry mediated through L-type channels enhances calcium release from sarcolemmal ryanodine receptors, allowing augmented calcium binding to troponin C. Conformational changes in the thin filament regulatory proteins allow more cross-bridge attachments between actin and myosin, with longer-lasting bonds and faster cycling of cross bridges (Figure 10). The result is a net increase in cardiac contractility without an increase in intracellular calcium concentration. Therefore,

Table 13: Nesiritide Dose (mg/kg/min)

Adverse Event	Control N=173	0.015 N=169	0.030 N=167	P value
Symptomatic hypotension	3%	8%	14%	0.003
Nausea	5%	10%	11%	0.092
Bradycardia	0%	4%	5%	0.003
Nervousness	0%	4%	1%	0.019

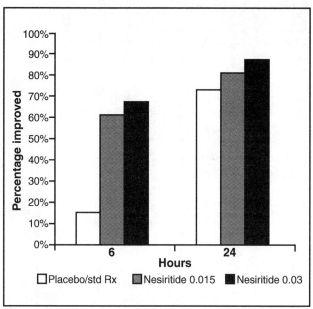

Figure 8: The effect of nesiritide on global clinical status/symptoms.

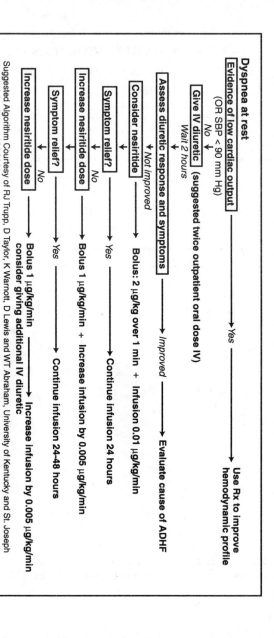

Figure 9: Treatment algorithm for 'wet' ADHF and use of nesiritide.

Dyspnea at rest
Evidence of low cardiac output
(OR SBP < 90 mm Hg)

No → Give IV diuretic (suggested twice outpatient oral dose IV)
Wait 2 hours

→ Assess diuretic response and symptoms

Yes → Use Rx to improve hemodynamic profile

Not improved → Consider nesiritide

Improved → Evaluate cause of ADHF

Symptom relief? → Bolus: 2 µg/kg over 1 min + Infusion 0.01 µg/kg/min

Yes → Continue infusion 24 hours

No → Increase nesiritide dose → Bolus 1 µg/kg/min + Increase infusion by 0.005 µg/kg/min

Symptom relief? Yes → Continue infusion 24-48 hours

No → Increase nesiritide dose → Bolus 1 µg/kg/min → Increase infusion by 0.005 µg/kg/min
consider giving additional IV diuretic

Suggested Algorithm Courtesy of RJ Trupp, D Taylor, K Warnott, D Lewis and WT Abraham, University of Kentucky and St. Joseph
Hospital, Lexington, KY, 2001.
OR = operating room; SBP = systolic blood pressure

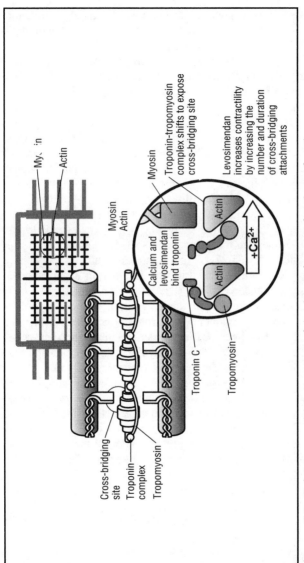

Figure 10: Calcium-sensitizing agents: levosimendan mechanism of action.

these agents may provide a more economical positive inotropic effect (ie, without a significant increase in myocardial oxygen consumption).

One such agent, levosimendan, has been compared with dobutamine in ADHF patients in double-blinded trials. The Levosimendan Infusion vs Dobutamine (LIDO) study evaluated the efficacy of treatment in achieving physician-predetermined goals for acute hemodynamic end points. Levosimendan was superior in this regard, with the treatment goal met in 28% of patients vs 15% of patients on dobutamine ($P=0.022$). Late evaluation of patient vitality revealed significantly improved survival in patients who had been treated with levosimendan at 30 and 180 days (Figure 11). The median number of patients alive and out of the hospital at 180 days after study drug administration was 157 for levosimendan-treated patients vs 133 for dobutamine-treated patients ($P=0.027$). A follow-up safety and efficacy study, the Randomized, Multicenter Evaluation of Intravenous Levosimendan Efficacy (REVIVE), is planned.

Endothelin (ET) antagonists inhibit the production of ET, another endogenous neurohormone with potent vasoconstrictor effects. ET levels increase in advanced heart failure and correlate with mortality risk. Increasing levels of angiotensin II, catecholamines, and insulin, as well as tissue shear stress, hypoxia, and other growth factors, stimulate ET production (Figure 12). ET synthesis is down-regulated by ANP, autocrine feedback, and vasodilatory prostaglandins. ET-1 is formed as a cleavage product of ET through ET-converting enzyme activity. Inhibition of the vasoconstrictor action of ET-1 may, therefore, be accomplished by inhibiting the converting enzyme and, consequently, ET formation or by blocking the site of action of ET on endothelial smooth muscle cells. Bosentan (Tracleer™), an oral ET-1 receptor blocker, has recently been approved for use in pulmonary arterial hypertension.

The Randomized Infusion of Tezosentan (RITZ) clinical trials 1 and 2 were conducted using an IV, nonselec-

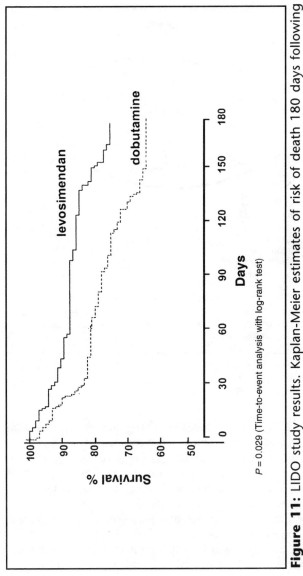

$P = 0.029$ (Time-to-event analysis with log-rank test)

Figure 11: LIDO study results. Kaplan-Meier estimates of risk of death 180 days following randomization.

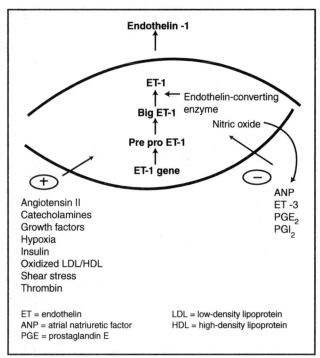

Figure 12: Formation of endothelin within the endothelial cell. Factors promoting formation and feedback inhibition.

tive ET antagonist, tezosentan. Together, the studies demonstrated that tezosentan was more effective than placebo at improving hemodynamics (higher cardiac index and lower pulmonary capillary wedge pressure) at 6 and 24 hours. At 6 hours, there was a dose-dependent increase in cardiac index between 24% and 50% vs 3% with placebo. No arrhythmia or hypotension requiring drug termination occurred. At 24 hours, the patient symptom score (dyspnea) was also significantly improved with tezosentan administration. Further trials with this agent are planned.

Discharge Planning

For most patients, this phase consists of 2 to 3 days of transition from IV diuretic and vasoactive medications to oral vasodilators and diuretics. Initiation of 'standard' medical therapy for heart failure or further up-titration of this regimen can be expedited by keeping the patient under close observation for side effects. The patient should begin to increase his or her daily activity level as tolerated. Continued evaluation and treatment of factors promoting acute decompensation is mandatory. When a history of patient noncompliance or failure to seek medical help early is a factor in precipitating rehospitalization, patient education and specific instruction are vital to the success of discharge planning and recidivism reduction. In the composite University Healthcare Consortium database, only 19% of 1,154 eligible heart failure patients received complete instructions on medications, diet, weight monitoring, activity, and what to do if symptoms worsen or recur and an appointment for medical follow-up (5% to 75%). Facilitating this transition helps make disease management programs successful.

Transitional Therapy

After hemodynamic stabilization and symptom alleviation, subsequent medical and ancillary interventions are intended to transition the stabilized patient toward discharge. This includes upward dose titration of oral vasodilators and diuretics with concomitant treatment of contributing comorbid conditions. Patient education about diagnosis, symptom recognition, and review of prescribed medications is critical to sustainable improvement. A rapid follow-up appointment (1 to 2 weeks) is an effective measure to avoid early readmission. Home-care nurse evaluation for compliance and in-home risk assessment while providing ongoing education are also helpful adjuncts. Figure 13 illustrates common reasons precipitating ADHF hospitalization, many of which are preventable with education and close follow-up. Unfortunately, the ancillary measures most of-

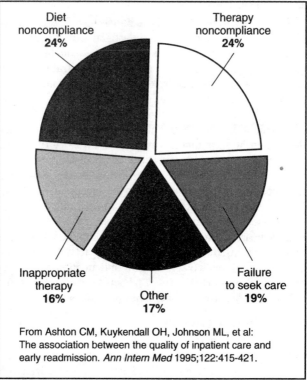

From Ashton CM, Kuykendall OH, Johnson ML, et al: The association between the quality of inpatient care and early readmission. *Ann Intern Med* 1995;122:415-421.

Figure 13: Common reasons for rehospitalization in chronic heart failure.

ten associated with good short-term outcome and low recidivism rates following discharge for ADHF are incomplete in 81% of hospitalizations (Figure 14).

Outpatient disease management programs provide highly cost-effective care for complex or refractory chronic heart failure patients, significantly reducing recurrent heart failure hospitalizations by up to 85%. The success of these programs is related to their accessibility and multifaceted approach to patient care emphasizing patient self-surveil-

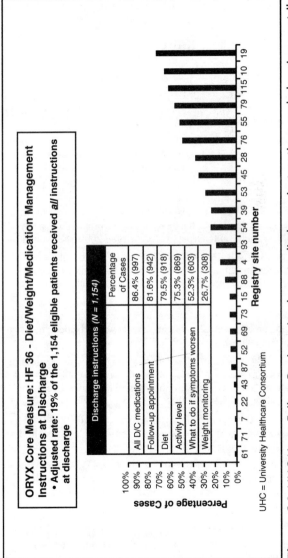

Figure 14: UHC Heart Failure Registry. Inadequate discharge instructions and planning contribute to recurrent hospitalizations.

239

lance and behavior modification through education and reinforcement of guideline-based medical therapy.

Suggested Readings

Adams KF Jr, Zannad F: Clinical definition and epidemiology of advanced heart failure. *Am Heart J* 1998;135:S204-S215.

Ashton CM, Kuykendall DH, Johnson ML, et al: The association between the quality of inpatient care and early readmission. *Ann Intern Med* 1995;122:415-421.

Chatterjee K, Hutchison SH, Chou TM: Acute ischemic heart failure: pathophysiology and management. In: Poole-Wilson PA, Colucci WS, Massie BM, eds. *Heart Failure. Scientific Principles and Clinical Practice*. New York, Churchill Livingstone, 1997, pp 523-549.

Colucci WS, Elkayam U, Horton DP, et al: Intravenous nesiritide, a natriuretic peptide, in the treatment of decompensated heart failure. Nesiritide Study Group. *N Engl J Med* 2000;343:246-253.

Cuffe MS, Califf RM, Adams KF Jr, et al: Short-term intravenous milrinone for acute exacerbation of heart failure: a randomized controlled trial. *JAMA* 2002;287:1541-1547.

Fonarow GC, Stevenson LW, Walden JA, et al: Impact of a comprehensive heart failure management program on hospital readmission and functional status of patients with advanced heart failure. *J Am Coll Cardiol* 1997;30:725-732.

Heart Failure Society of America (HFSA) practice guidelines. HFSA guidelines for management of patients with heart failure caused by left ventricular systolic dysfunction—pharmacological approaches. *J Card Fail* 1999;5:357-382.

Hermann DD, Greenberg BH: Refractory heart failure: beyond standard therapy. In: Sharpe N, ed. *Heart Failure Management*. London, Martin Dunitz Ltd, 2000, pp 199-216.

Hunt SA, Baker DW, Chin MH, et al: ACC/AHA guidelines for the evaluation and management of chronic heart failure in the adult. A report of the American College of Cardiology/American Heart Association Task Force on Practice Guidelines (Committee to Revise the 1995 Guidelines for the Evaluation and Management of Heart Failure). *J Am Coll Cardiol* 2001;38:2101-2113. Full text available at http://www.acc.org/clinical/guidelines/failure/hf_index.htm.

Intravenous nesiritide vs nitroglycerin for treatment of decompensated congestive heart failure: a randomized controlled trial. *JAMA* 2002;287:1531-1540.

Krumholz HM, Parent EM, Tu N, et al: Readmission after hospitalization for congestive heart failure among Medicare beneficiaries. *Arch Intern Med* 1997;157:99-104.

Leier CV, Binkley PF: Parenteral inotropic support for advanced congestive heart failure. *Prog Cardiovasc Dis* 1998;41:207-224.

Lubsen J, Just H, Hjalmarsson AC, et al: Effect of pimobendan on exercise capacity in patients with heart failure: main results from the Pimobendan in Congestive Heart Failure (PICO) trial. *Heart* 1996;76:223-231.

Mills RM, LeJemtel TH, Horton DP, et al: Sustained hemodynamic effects of an infusion of nesiritide (human b-type natriuretic peptide) in heart failure: a randomized, double-blind, placebo-controlled trial. Natrecor Study Group. *J Am Coll Cardiol* 1999;34:155-162.

Mueller HS, Chatterjee K, Davis KB, et al: ACC expert consensus document. Present use of bedside right heart catheterization in patients with cardiac disease. American College of Cardiology. *J Am Coll Cardiol* 1998;32:840-864.

Niemenen MS, Akkila J, Hasenfuss G, et al: Hemodynamic and neurohumoral effects of continuous infusion of levosimendan in patients with congestive heart failure. *J Am Coll Cardiol* 2000;36:1903-1912.

Packer M, Carver JR, Rodeheffer RJ, et al: Effect of oral milrinone on mortality in severe chronic heart failure. The PROMISE Study Research Group. *N Engl J Med* 1991;325:1468-1475.

Richenbacher WE, Pierce WS: Assisted circulation and the mechanical heart. In: Braunwald E, ed. *Heart Disease. A Textbook on Cardiovascular Medicine*. Philadelphia, WB Saunders, 1997, pp 534-547.

Rubin LJ, Badesch DB, Barst RJ, et al: Bosentan therapy for pulmonary arterial hypertension. *N Engl J Med* 2002;346:896-903.

Steimle AE, Warner-Stevenson LW, Chelimsky-Fallick C, et al: Sustained hemodynamic efficacy of therapy tailored to reduce filling pressures in survivors with advanced heart failure. *Circulation* 1997;96:1165-1172.

Stevenson LW: Inotropic therapy for heart failure. *N Engl J Med* 1998;339:1848-1850.

Stevenson LW, Massie BM, Francis GS, et al: Optimizing therapy for complex or refractory heart failure: a management algorithm. *Am Heart J* 1998;135:S293-S309.

Torre-Amione G, Young JB, Durand J, et al: Hemodynamic effects of tezosentan, an intravenous dual endothelin receptor antagonist, in patients with class III to IV congestive heart failure. *Circulation* 2001;103:973-980.

Trupp RJ, Taylor D, Warnott K, et al: *Natrecor Algorithm Contributors*. Lexington, KY, University of Kentucky and St. Joseph Hospital, 2001.

Chapter **8**

Treatment of Chronic Heart Failure

The treatment of chronic heart failure has evolved substantially during the past 2 decades. As recently as 20 years ago, there were few successful options for medical treatment beyond the mainstays of digoxin (Lanoxin®) and diuretics. Bed rest, often for prolonged periods, was still recommended for some patients, and vasodilator therapy had only just emerged. Moreover, although the available therapeutic options were effective in providing relief of symptoms, these approaches did little to alter the natural history of heart failure. As a result, morbidity and mortality remained high. The future for patients diagnosed with heart failure during this era was not bright.

During the past 20 years, in tandem with important insights into the underlying pathophysiology of cardiac dysfunction, powerful new approaches to heart failure treatment have been developed. The drugs that have been introduced into the therapeutic regimen not only provide symptomatic relief, but also have a substantial impact on the natural history of heart failure. Patients with heart failure who are treated with these agents feel better and live longer. Additionally, the aggressive application of new therapies has been shown to not only inhibit the progressive deterioration in cardiac function characteristic of heart failure, but also reverse the structural and functional changes in the heart in many patients. Thus, in the first decade of the new millennium, heart failure diagnosis is no longer the death sentence that it has been in the past. We now have many reasons to be optimistic about the outcome of patients with this condition.

This chapter summarizes the approach to managing patients with chronic heart failure, extending from prevention of heart failure to management of patients with severe refractory disease. In this chapter (as throughout the book), the preferred term is *heart failure* rather than *congestive heart failure*. The difference is more than semantic, since the terms developed parallel to our understanding of the pathophysiology of the condition, and many patients may have heart failure without being congested.

Natural History

Heart failure is a clinical syndrome and, as such, can result from a wide variety of underlying diseases. This chapter examines chronic heart failure caused by systolic dysfunction of the heart. Table 1 lists some of the common causes of this condition. Most heart failure in the United States and other industrialized countries is caused by hypertension and/or coronary artery disease (CAD). In each case, damage to the heart initiates the process of progressive remodeling that leads to ever-worsening cardiac function. This process is described in greater detail in Chapter 1.

Most often, cardiac remodeling and progressive deterioration in cardiac function take place over an extended period. This delay affords opportunities for intervention that can inhibit and even reverse the process that underlies heart failure. However, all too often, the threat to the patient is not fully recognized and therapy is not initiated until after the clinical manifestations of heart failure appear. Even then, initiation of optimal therapy may be unduly delayed, and the patient remains at risk of further

Table 1: Major Causes of Heart Failure in the United States

- Coronary artery disease/myocardial infarction
- Hypertension
- Valvular heart disease
- Infections (eg, viral myocarditis, Chagas disease, HIV)
- Myocardial toxins (eg, doxorubicin [Adriamycin®], trastuzumab [Herceptin®], alcohol, cocaine, methamphetamines)
- Infiltrative disease (eg, sarcoidosis, amyloidosis, hemochromatosis)
- Tachycardia
- Hyperthyroidism/hypothyroidism
- Peripartum
- Familial
- Pericardial disease
- Congenital heart lesions

progression of the underlying disease, as well as the attendant morbidity and mortality associated with heart failure. This is unfortunate because initiation of optimal therapy for heart failure, such as the use of neurohormonal blocking agents, has been associated with >50% reduction in annualized mortality risk.

Despite these advances, however, heart failure remains a lethal condition. Patients with New York Heart Association (NYHA) Class IV symptoms of heart failure have an expected annual mortality of 20% to 50%. Patients with milder NYHA Class II-III symptoms still have an annual mortality rate of 10% to 15%. Even patients with asymp-

Table 2: Common Causes of Worsening Heart Failure

- Medical noncompliance
- Dietary indiscretion
- Intercurrent infection
- Comorbidities (eg, renal failure, hepatic or pulmonary disease)
- Myocardial ischemia
- Anemia
- Rhythm abnormalities (most commonly atrial tachyarrhythmias)
- Chronotropic incompetence and/or heart block
- Hyperthyroidism/hypothyroidism
- Sleep apnea

tomatic left ventricular (LV) dysfunction are at increased risk of dying; they have an annual mortality rate in the range of 5%. Overall, approximately 50% of heart failure patients are likely to die within 5 years, a mortality rate that compares unfavorably with most malignancies. These figures are a reminder that complacency should be avoided when the therapeutic approach to the patient with heart failure is being considered, even when patients appear clinically well compensated and without fluid overload.

Worsening Heart Failure

Heart failure is a chronic disease, and the clinical course may extend over many years. Consequently, it is not surprising that during the course of the disease, patients will present one or (usually) more times with decompensated heart failure. With each episode of decompensation, the question of whether it was caused by deterioration in un-

Table 3: Causes of Medical Noncompliance

- Inadequate understanding of the rationale for the medical regimen
- Difficulty in refilling prescriptions
- Physical limitations in taking multiple drugs throughout the day (eg, arthritis, orthopedic conditions, visual impairment)
- Failure to understand dosing regimen(s)
- Inability to afford the drugs
- Side effects (real or not)
- General 'ornery' and recalcitrant disposition of the patient

derlying LV performance as opposed to the interposition of a temporary and often remediable cause should be raised. Early identification of a correctable cause of decompensated heart failure is an important goal of the evaluation of patients who present with worsening signs and symptoms, since this information can have profound effects on the subsequent management and clinical course. Table 2 lists common conditions associated with worsening heart failure.

The most common cause of decompensation or worsening heart failure is the failure of patients to comply with the therapeutic regimen. The reasons for this are numerous; some of the more common ones are outlined in Table 3. A unifying trend in many of these situations is poor communication between the patient and the health-care team. Possible reasons for this problem are listed in Table 4.

One approach to solving this problem is the development of an organized heart failure program staffed by a dedicated team of health professionals who are experi-

Table 4: Possible Reasons for Poor Communication Between the Medical Team and the Patient

- Educational, language, or cultural differences between the patient and the health-care team
- Information regarding heart failure given while the patient is hospitalized and/or acutely ill
- Lack of reinforcement of the message
- Failure to educate the spouse (or significant other) as well as the patient

enced in managing heart failure patients. The success of these programs in improving the clinical course of heart failure patients has been well documented in medical literature. These programs have proven to be a cost-effective way of managing large groups of patients with heart failure. Much of their success is related to their ability to improve patient compliance and heighten patient (and family) awareness of the early warning signs of worsening heart failure. This, in turn, allows the patient to initiate changes in therapy (eg, increased diuretic doses) that circumvent more serious episodes of decompensation.

Prevention of Heart Failure

Interventions that effectively reduce the likelihood of heart failure are outlined in Table 5. As mentioned previously, most heart failure in the United States and other industrialized countries develops as a consequence of CAD and/or hypertension, and a history of hypertension continues to be associated with heart failure in approximately 75% of patients. A review of recent, large-scale clinical trials of new therapies for heart failure indicates that 60% to 80% of patients with heart failure caused by systolic

Table 5: Primary Prevention of Heart Failure

- Treatment of hypercholesterolemia
- Treatment of hypertension (diastolic and isolated systolic hypertension)
- Aspirin treatment in patients with coronary disease
- Use of angiotensin-converting enzyme (ACE) inhibitors in patients who are post-MI or at risk* for coronary events
- Use of β-blockers post-MI
- Use of ACE inhibitors in patients with asymptomatic LV dysfunction
- Use of angiotensin-receptor blockers (ARBs) in patients with diabetes and evidence of renal dysfunction

*Patients with evidence of coronary, cerebral, or peripheral artery disease, and patients with diabetes and one additional risk factor (eg, smoking, hypercholesterolemia, hypertension).

dysfunction had an ischemic etiology as the cause. It stands to reason that interventions that effectively treat hypertension and CAD should have an important impact on the future risk of heart failure. Now, there is convincing evidence that this is the case. Treatment of high blood pressure in the Systolic Hypertension in the Elderly Population (SHEP) and the Swedish Trial in Old Patients (STOP) studies demonstrated significant reductions in cardiovascular disease. Researchers found that the risk of heart failure was lowered to 50%, a reduction that was greater than that for any other cardiovascular condition. Hypercholesterolemia is a well-recognized risk factor for CAD, and treatment of this condition with statins has been shown to significantly reduce the likelihood of cardiovascular events and to improve survival. The results of the Scandinavian Simvastatin Survival Study (4S) indicate that the risk of heart failure was also significantly reduced by simvastatin (Zocor®). The striking results of these studies substantiate the concept that treatment of risk factors will have a highly significant impact on preventing heart failure in the future.

The Heart Outcomes Prevention Evaluation (HOPE) study was designed to assess the effects of prophylactic angiotensin-converting enzyme (ACE) inhibitor treatment of patients with either manifest atherosclerotic disease or high risk of it on a variety of cardiovascular end points. The study showed that after 5 years, patients who received the ACE inhibitor ramipril (Altace®) had a significant reduction in a composite end point of stroke, nonfatal myocardial infarction (MI), or death because of cardiovascular cause. Each component of this composite was also significantly reduced by ramipril. Not surprisingly, the risk of heart failure hospitalization was also reduced by ACE inhibitor therapy in the HOPE study. These results provide convincing evidence that patients with coronary, cerebral, or peripheral vascular disease (or who have diabetes and other risk factors) should be receiving an ACE inhibitor. The results of HOPE are more fully examined in Chapter 4.

The Reduction of Endpoints in Non-Insulin Dependent Diabetes Mellitus with the Angiotensin II Antagonist Losartan (RENAAL) study assessed the impact of the angiotensin-receptor blocker (ARB) losartan (Cozaar®, Hyzaar®) in patients with type II diabetes and evidence of renal involvement. Approximately 92% of the patients also had hypertension. The study demonstrated that adding losartan to the medical regimen reduced the risk of worsening renal disease in this population. Again, there was a reduction in the risk of developing heart failure in the RENAAL population that was treated with losartan.

Treatment of Asymptomatic Left Ventricular Dysfunction

As described in Chapter 1, damage to the heart sets in motion a complex series of events resulting in progressive remodeling of the left ventricle. Overall, there are increases in cardiac chamber volume and muscle mass and conformational changes in the left ventricle. The net effect of these changes is the development of systolic and diastolic dysfunction of the heart. Often, the process goes on unrecognized for years before overt heart failure becomes manifest. Some of the factors involved in the remodeling process have been identified, and early treatment has been shown to effectively block the structural changes in the heart and the progression to heart failure.

One of the most important insights into heart failure pathophysiology that has emerged over the past decades is the role of neurohormonal activation in promoting progression of disease. This issue is examined more fully in Chapter 1 and in the chapters reviewing the use of drugs to block the renin-angiotensin-aldosterone system and the use of β-blockers (Chapters 4 and 5). Treatment of patients with LV dysfunction who are at risk of developing heart failure combines risk factor management approaches to inhibit/reverse further remodeling of the heart. Recommendations for therapy of asymptomatic LV dysfunction are included in Table 5.

The effects of treating asymptomatic LV dysfunction with an ACE inhibitor were evaluated in the prevention arm of the Studies of Left Ventricular Dysfunction (SOLVD). The results demonstrated that administration of enalapril (Lexxel®, Vasotec®) to patients with an LV ejection fraction (LVEF) <0.35 reduced future risk of heart failure and heart failure-related events. In this study, adding the ACE inhibitor to the medical regimen reduced the combined end point of death or heart failure hospitalization by 20% ($P<0.001$). Moreover, the rate of progression from the asymptomatic state to overt heart failure was substantially prolonged by the prophylactic use of an ACE inhibitor. The development of heart failure was reduced by 37%, and the likelihood of heart failure hospitalization was reduced by 44% (both $P<0.001$). An echocardiographic substudy of SOLVD showed that the beneficial effects of enalapril were at least partially related to the effects of ACE inhibition in attenuating the progressive remodeling of the left ventricle that was seen in the placebo-treated SOLVD patients.

The use of ACE inhibitors and β-blockers has also been shown to benefit MI survivors with a reduced EF but without evidence of heart failure. In the Survival and Ventricular Enlargement (SAVE) trial, MI survivors with an EF <0.40 were randomized to captopril or placebo. The group receiving captopril experienced a significant 19% reduction in mortality ($P=0.019$) and a significant 37% reduction in the onset of heart failure. In the Carvedilol Post-Infarct Survival Control in Left Ventricular Dysfunction (CAPRICORN) trial, post-MI patients with an EF <0.40 who were randomized to the β-blocker carvedilol (Coreg®) experienced a significant 23% reduction in mortality compared to a placebo group. Nonfatal MI was significantly reduced in the carvedilol-treated patients, and the combined risk of death and nonfatal MI was reduced by 41%. The CAPRICORN study is of particular importance because it assesses the benefits of post-MI β-blocker therapy in the modern interventional era. Patients enrolled in CAPRICORN were also already receiving an ACE inhibitor, so the results demonstrate the added benefit of giving carvedilol to post-MI patients with LV dysfunction. When considered together, these trials suggest that the combination of an ACE inhibitor and β-blocker in post-MI patients with a low EF result in a reduction of mortality in the range of 40%. Needless to say, there is also a substantial reduction in the risk of developing heart failure in this population.

Table 6: Goals of Therapy for Heart Failure

- Alleviate symptoms of congestion
- Improve tissue perfusion
- Increase exercise capacity
- Improve quality of life
- Prevent or reverse progressive cardiac dysfunction
- Improve survival
- Reduce hospitalizations

Treatment of Patients With Mild-Moderate Heart Failure

The presence of heart failure is often first detected when the patient presents with symptoms related to fluid retention and/or fatigue. Even with treatment, however, most patients with heart failure continue to have mild-moderate symptoms or limitation in their exercise capacity. Thus, 60% to 70% of the heart failure population would be considered to have NYHA Class II-III symptoms of heart failure.

The goals of therapy in this group of patients are outlined in Table 6. In broad terms, they include alleviating symptoms, preventing progression of the underlying disease, and reducing morbidity and mortality. Whereas 20 years ago, only the former would have been possible, there is now convincing evidence that aggressive use of neurohormonal blocking agents will effectively inhibit progression of LV dysfunction and, in some cases, reverse the underlying disease process. This, in turn, has been associated with improved survival and diminished rate of hospitalization. As in patients who are either at risk of developing LV dysfunction or have asymptom-

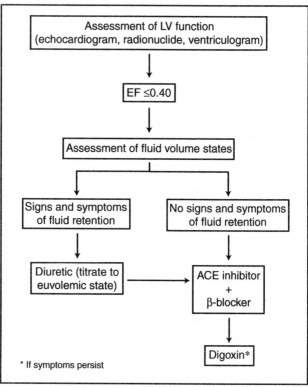

Figure 1: An overview of managing patients with mild-moderate heart failure. Consensus recommendations for the management of chronic heart failure. On behalf of the membership of the advisory council to improve outcomes nationwide in heart failure. *Am J Cardiol* 1999; 83(suppl 2A):1A-38A. These recommendations have been slightly modified by the authors.

atic dysfunction, prevention of further damage or progression of disease is an important goal. Thus, the strategies that are outlined in Table 5 should also be used in patients with symptomatic disease.

Table 7: Use of Diuretics to Treat Chronic Heart Failure

- Loop diuretics are preferred because of greater diuretic potency and less potassium wasting.

- Potassium and magnesium levels must be checked at regular intervals to determine the need for replacement therapy.

- Increased diuretic requirements during an episode of decompensated heart failure may not be needed after the patient returns to baseline, particularly if a correctable cause for the deterioration can be identified.

- Although diuretics are needed to alleviate signs/symptoms of fluid retention, they may increase activation of the renin-angiotensin system.

Table 8: Side Effects of Diuretic Therapy

- Hypokalemia
- Hypomagnesemia
- Hyperuricemia and gout
- Hyperglycemia
- Increased plasma renin activity
- Overdiuresis resulting in decreased cardiac output and diminished tissue perfusion

An overview of managing patients with mild-moderate heart failure is shown in Figure 1; the approach to diagnosis is reviewed in Chapter 2. However, it is important to stress that measuring the LVEF at the time that heart failure is first recognized is essential for the rational planning of further management. Since most patients with systolic dysfunction either present with or develop fluid retention at some point during the course of their illness, diuretic agents are an essential component of the management of symptomatic heart failure. Loop diuretics (ie, furosemide [Lasix®], bumetanide [Bumex®], torsemide [Demadex®], or ethacrynic acid [Edecrin®]) are preferred in treating heart failure patients based on their potency in promoting salt and water loss and the lesser amount of potassium wasting compared to thiazide diuretics. The use of diuretic agents is examined in greater detail in Chapter 3. Some aspects of the use of diuretics that are helpful in outpatient management of heart failure are listed in Table 7. Although generally well tolerated, diuretics are not without side effects. Some common problems that may result from diuretic therapy are outlined in Table 8.

The goal of diuretic therapy is to reduce filling pressures within the heart to alleviate the signs and symptoms of congestion while maintaining adequate cardiac output. Although there is little to indicate that diuretic agents improve systolic pump function by bringing the heart back from a descending limb of the Frank-Starling curve, diuresis may actually result in improved cardiac output in many instances. This is probably related to decreased afterload and a reduction in myocardial ischemia as the ventricle is reduced in size. Diuresis may also reduce the peripheral vasoconstriction that acts to impede LV emptying by decreasing the intense neurohormonal activation that accompanies decompensated heart failure. Perhaps the most potent factor in diuretic-related increases in cardiac output is that reduction in cardiac chamber size with diuresis improves the competence of the mitral valve and reduces the amount of mitral regurgitation. This results in a redirection of mitral regurgitant flow toward more useful forward cardiac output.

One of the most important issues in determining the appropriate dose of diuretics is that 'overdiuresis' can have the unintended consequence of further compromising cardiac output when filling pressures are reduced beyond an optimal level. This is usually manifested by one or more of the signs of hypoperfusion, such as a reduction in arterial pressure (resulting in lightheadedness or presyncope) or a rise in renal function parameters. In this case, the increase in blood urea nitrogen (BUN) often exceeds the creatinine so that the patient develops a pattern consistent with prerenal azotemia.

As outlined in Chapter 4, all patients with symptomatic heart failure caused by LV systolic dysfunction should be treated with an ACE inhibitor. These agents have been shown to improve survival by 20% in patients with mild-moderate heart failure and to reduce hospitalizations. Dosing of ACE inhibitors in heart failure and issues related to side effects are outlined in depth in Chapter 4.

Despite abundant evidence for the efficacy of ACE inhibitors in treating heart failure, there is still evidence that they are underused and underdosed. The major reason for this is the physician's concern about the blood pressure level at the initiation and up-titration phase. However, in the opinion of most heart failure experts, this is much less of a limiting factor than might be expected. A useful rule of thumb is that evidence of hypoperfusion, not the absolute level of blood pressure, should dictate the titration of the ACE inhibitor. Thus, even blood pressures of 80 mm Hg (or below) should not be used as a reason to withhold therapy or keep the dose at a low level if there is no evidence of lightheadedness or a rise in renal function tests indicating compromised renal perfusion. Some increase in renal function tests is to be expected with the initiation of ACE inhibitors even in patients with higher levels of blood pressure. Importantly, this reflects a functional and usually reversible effect rather than a structural and irreversible change in the kidney.

Two side effects of ACE inhibitors that may require discontinuation are ACE inhibitor-induced cough and angioedema. When a severe cough or angioedema occurs, the ACE inhibitor should be discontinued and the patient switched to an alternative therapy, such as an ARB. Although cough should not occur with the ARBs, angioedema has been reported with these agents and some caution is advisable in initiating them, particularly if the ACE inhibitor-induced angioedema involved compromised air movement.

As shown in the Valsartan in Heart Failure Trial (Val-HeFT), the addition of an ARB to an ACE inhibitor reduces the combined end point of mortality/morbidity by 13% in heart failure patients. This significant reduction occurs because of an impact on heart failure hospitalizations, which are reduced by 27% compared to use of an ACE inhibitor alone. There is no effect, however, of the ACE inhibitor/ARB combination on mortality. Since subgroup analysis of Val-HeFT results suggested that those patients on either an ACE inhibitor or β-blocker alone were most likely to improve, an ARB should be considered for patients who cannot tolerate an ACE inhibitor or a β-blocker. There was also a suggestion that the combination of a β-blocker, ACE inhibitor, and ARB was associated with increased risk in Val-HeFT. Thus, until further study, the addition of an ARB to a patient already receiving an ACE inhibitor and a β-blocker should be avoided.

The rationale, results, and methods of using β-blockers in heart failure are outlined in Chapter 5. The considerable benefits of β-blockade in patients with mild-moderate heart failure have now been demonstrated in several large-scale clinical trials. As a result, β-blockers have emerged over the past few years as a standard of therapy for patients with this condition. The addition of β-blockers to the medical regimen can be expected to reduce mortality by 35%, reduce hospitalizations significantly, improve symptoms and quality of life, and increase EF. Moreover, these benefits are additive to those caused by ACE inhibitors. Administering these agents together produces >50% reduction in mortality.

β-blockers should not be started while the patient remains 'wet'—they should be initiated after diuretics and ACE inhibitors have been begun and the patient no longer has signs or symptoms of volume overload. Although most experts in the field start a β-blocker after an ACE inhibitor (which is usually begun at the time that diuretics are started), there is no reason why the order cannot be reversed in euvolemic patients who are not on an ACE inhibitor. Failure to initiate and up-titrate a β-blocker is often caused by the same concern about blood pressure as with ACE inhibitor therapy. Again, recommendations for β-blocker treatment are based on presence of hypoperfusion rather than on the level of blood pressure per se. An examination of the practical aspects of β-blocker therapy can be found in Chapter 5.

A common question regarding the management of patients with mild-moderate heart failure is whether there is still a role for digoxin in patients who are in sinus rhythm. Digoxin's use in the atrial fibrillation setting is secure based on its effects in helping maintain rate control. The results of large-scale digoxin trials failed to demonstrate any evidence that digoxin has either a favorable or an unfavorable effect on survival in heart failure patients in normal sinus rhythm. However, the study did demonstrate that patients remaining on digoxin experienced a 10% reduction in hospitalization, an effect that confirmed the favorable effects of digoxin seen in smaller trials with this agent. The Prospective Randomized Study of Ventricular Failure and the Efficacy of Digoxin (PROVED) and Randomized Assessment of Digoxin and Inhibitors of Angiotensin-Converting Enzyme (RADIANCE) studies also reported increased exercise capacity and symptomatic improvement in patients who were not withdrawn from digoxin. Thus, digoxin is recommended for patients who remain symptomatic despite therapy with diuretics, ACE inhibitors, and β-blockers.

Aspirin is also commonly used in heart failure patients. The rationale for this is that most heart failure patients have underlying CAD and the use of aspirin has been shown to favorably affect the outcome in this setting. The other advantage is that patients with heart failure are at risk of developing thrombi within the chambers of the heart, and the subsequent embolization can be an important cause of morbidity and mortality in this population. Whether aspirin can prevent thrombus formation in patients with heart failure, however, is uncertain. Additionally, there is some evidence that aspirin may reduce the efficacy of ACE inhibitor therapy, probably by blocking release of prostaglandins and other substances that are stimulated by the ACE inhibitor-induced increase in bradykinin. Nonetheless, most experts agree that aspirin is warranted in patients with heart failure. Some would, however, give 81 mg daily to patients with nonischemic etiology of their heart failure and reserve the higher 325-mg dose for patients with a history or evidence of CAD.

The question of whether to treat heart failure patients with warfarin (Coumadin®) is controversial. Clearly, warfarin is indicated in patients with atrial fibrillation to prevent thromboembolic complications. A retrospective analysis of the SOLVD study also suggested that patients treated with warfarin had better survival than those who were not treated with this agent. Thus, some heart failure experts recommend coumadinization for patients in sinus rhythm, particularly if the EF is severely depressed. Others (including the authors) favor a more conservative approach, reserving anticoagulation therapy for patients with a history of thromboemboli, demonstration of a clot within the heart by echocardiogram, or the presence of 'smoke' (an indicator of low cardiac output and stasis within the heart) on echocardiogram.

Treatment of Severe or Refractory Heart Failure

Patients who remain symptomatic at rest or with mild exertion despite optimal treatment with the drugs outlined

Table 9: Drugs/Approaches for Treating Severe or Refractory Heart Failure

- Spironolactone (Aldactone®)
- Non-ACE inhibitor vasodilators (ie, hydralazine nitrates)
- Addition of metolazone (Zaroxolyn®, Mykrox®) to a loop diuretic
- Admission for 'tailored' therapy
- Outpatient inotrope therapy
- Cardiac transplantation
- LV assist device (LVAD)

are considered to have severe heart failure. The term *refractory* usually implies that they remain volume overloaded despite intensive diuretic therapy. Thus, these patients are at high risk for death and/or hospitalization, and an aggressive therapeutic approach is indicated. Once reversible causes of decompensation have been excluded, additional approaches and therapies can be enlisted (Table 9).

Most patients with refractory heart failure have evidence of fluid overload despite intensive diuretic therapy. Diuretic resistance because of renal tubular cell hypertrophy is a well-described phenomenon in patients with heart failure and plays an important role in developing refractory heart failure. Reductions in renal blood flow caused by low cardiac output or renal perfusion pressure (sometimes related to overaggressive treatment with diuretics, neurohormonal blockers, or vasodilators) may also be involved in some cases of diuretic resistance. When increases in the loop diuretic dose fail to produce adequate diuresis, the addition of a second diuretic that acts on another segment of the nephron is often used. An agent such as metolazone (Mykrox®,

Zaroxolyn®), which acts on the distal portion of the nephron, is often chosen. Although this combined approach is an effective way of increasing diuresis, it should be used sparingly because of the potent electrolyte wasting effects. In particular, this combination leads to increased excretion of potassium and magnesium, and unless this is carefully monitored and deficiencies are corrected, the patient will be at risk for developing hypokalemia and hypomagnesemia, which are associated with potentially fatal ventricular arrhythmias. Additionally, when the combination of metolazone and a loop diuretic is continued after the patient has regained an euvolemic state, there is the possibility of 'overdiuresing.' This can lead to a reduction in blood pressure, inadequate renal blood flow, and evidence of worsening renal function. Thus, patients in whom metolazone has been added should be followed closely with careful assessment of volume status to determine when and if the second diuretic can be reduced or discontinued. However, some patients will require maintenance of combined diuretic therapy as part of their treatment to maintain an euvolemic state.

The benefits and approach to the addition of spironolactone (Aldactone®) and non-ACE inhibitor vasodilators are described in Chapters 3 and 4. Spironolactone has been shown in the Randomized Aldactone Evaluation Study (RALES) trial to reduce all-cause mortality by 30% when added to standard therapy, such as ACE inhibitors, in patients with advanced heart failure.

Non-ACE inhibitor vasodilators refer to the use of nonparenteral nitrates, usually in combination with hydralazine. Although both agents are vasodilators and can acutely improve cardiac hemodynamic variables, there is some evidence that the main benefit of hydralazine is to prevent tolerance to the nitrate. The combination of hydralazine and a long-acting nitrate has been shown to reduce mortality in heart failure patients in the Veterans Administration Heart Failure Trial I (V-HeFT I). However, ACE inhibitors were shown to be more effective in this regard in V-HeFT II. This fact, as well as the difficulties in compliance with the hydralazine/nitrate combination, has relegated this therapy to second-line use in patients who are unable to tolerate an ACE inhibitor or ARB. However, in the experience of many heart failure experts, the hydralazine/nitrate combination can improve symptoms in otherwise refractory patients. Improved exercise capacity in heart failure patients has also been demonstrated with long-acting nitrate preparations. Both agents have been shown to favorably affect the pattern of blood flow within the heart in patients with mitral regurgitation. Since secondary mitral regurgitation is commonly seen in patients with advanced heart failure, the hydralazine/nitrate combination provides a means of reducing regurgitant flow and improving cardiac performance in patients with this condition.

Tailored therapy is an approach that involves the use of hemodynamic monitoring with a balloon-tipped right heart catheter to help guide drug administration. This procedure necessitates hospitalization in an ICU setting and should be reserved for patients who fail to respond to more conventional approaches and who are markedly limited by symptoms of heart failure. It can also be used in patients in whom there is a real question about the severity of the symptoms or in whom there is discordance between objective signs and subjective complaints. With hemodynamic guidance doses of diuretics, both ACE inhibitors and non-ACE inhibitor vasodilator drugs can be optimized. Often, a short course of inotropic agents or intravenous (IV) vasodilators is used to help facilitate the process. Experts in the field report substantial improvement with this approach, and the results of tailored therapy are now being critically assessed in a large-scale clinical trial.

The use of inotropic agents in the treatment of acute decompensated heart failure and a description of the agents can be found in Chapter 7. Although there is a paucity of information available describing long-term

Table 10: Indications for Cardiac Transplantation

- Refractory heart failure despite optimal medical therapy
- Risk factors indicative of poor survival (eg, extremely low EF, markedly diminished exercise capacity, recurrent hospitalizations)
- Refractory ventricular arrhythmias
- Severe ischemic heart disease without potential for revascularization and refractory angina or heart failure
- Congenital or valvular heart disease not amenable to surgical repair
- Giant cell myocarditis
- Absence of noncardiac disease that would reduce expected survival to less than 5 years
- Good psychosocial support system

results, outpatient IV inotropic therapy appears to have some value for patients who are truly refractory and cannot leave the hospital without this treatment. It is also used in patients awaiting cardiac transplantation who cannot be maintained on oral medications alone. In such patients, the optimal dose is established while they are in the hospital, using guidance with a right heart catheter. A long-term indwelling venous catheter is placed, and the patient is discharged on either continuous or intermittent therapy. The advantage of this approach compared to intermittent therapy in an outpatient clinic is that it avoids frequent and lengthy trips to the clinic or infusion center. The disadvantage of therapy in the outpatient setting is that immediate treatment of drug-related side effects, such as arrhythmia or hypotension,

Table 11: Exclusions for Cardiac Transplantation

- Irreversible renal failure
- Fixed, severe pulmonary hypertension
- Diabetes with severe end-organ damage
- Continued substance abuse (ie, alcohol, tobacco, illegal drugs)
- Infections with hepatitis B and C with biopsy evidence of liver disease
- Liver disease with total bilirubin >3.0
- Chronic obstructive airway disease with an FEV_1 <1 L
- Active chronic infection (eg, chronic sinusitis, otitis media, bronchiectasis with resistant organisms)
- HIV infection
- Severe debilitation
- Noncompliance

cannot be undertaken. In many cases, outpatient inotropic therapy produces considerable symptomatic relief and reduces hospitalizations. The terminally ill patient has an opportunity to live outside of the hospital in the last stages of his or her illness.

Role of Cardiac Transplantation

Cardiac transplantation is now an established treatment for patients with severe refractory heart failure. Survival after cardiac transplantation has gotten progressively better over the years because of the availability of more effective immunosuppressive agents to treat posttransplantation rejection. At the University of California, San Diego, 1-

and 5-year posttransplant survival rates are 93% and 81%, respectively. Given the high expected mortality in the patients who were transplanted, this represents a substantial improvement in the clinical course. Thus, cardiac transplantation should be considered for patients with severe symptomatic limitation or high risk of mortality. Indications and major exclusions for cardiac transplantation are outlined in Tables 10 and 11.

Suggested Readings

Al-Khadra AS, Salem DN, Rand WM, et al: Antiplatelet agents and survival: a cohort analysis from the Studies of Left Ventricular Dysfunction (SOLVD) trial. *J Am Coll Cardiol* 1998;31:419-425.

Bristow MR: β-adrenergic receptor blockade in chronic heart failure. *Circulation* 2000;101:558-569.

The Cardiac Insufficiency Bisoprolol Study II (CIBIS-II): a randomized trial. *Lancet* 1999;353:9-13.

Cohn JN, Archibald DG, Ziesche S, et al: Effect of vasodilator therapy on mortality in chronic congestive heart failure. Results of a Veterans Administration Cooperative Study. *N Engl J Med* 1986;314:1547-1552.

Cohn JN, Johnson G, Ziesche S, et al: A comparison of enalapril with hydralazine-isosorbide dinitrate in the treatment of chronic congestive heart failure. *N Engl J Med* 1991;325:303-310.

Consensus recommendations for the management of chronic heart failure. On behalf of the membership of the advisory council to improve outcomes nationwide in heart failure. *Am J Cardiol* 1999;83:1A-38A.

Costantini O, Huck K, Carlson MD, et al: Impact of a guideline-based disease management team on outcomes of hospitalized patients with congestive heart failure. *Arch Intern Med* 2001;161:177-182.

Doughty RN, Whalley GA, Gamble G, et al: Left ventricular remodeling with carvedilol in patients with congestive heart failure due to ischemic heart disease. Australia-New Zealand Heart Failure Research Collaborative Group. *J Am Coll Cardiol* 1997; 29:1060-1066.

The effect of digoxin on mortality and morbidity in patients with heart failure. The Digitalis Investigation Group. *N Engl J Med* 1997;336:525-533.

Effect of enalapril on mortality and the development of heart failure in asymptomatic patients with reduced left ventricular ejection fractions. The SOLVD Investigators. *N Engl J Med* 1992;327:685-691.

Effect of enalapril on survival in patients with reduced left ventricular ejection fractions and congestive heart failure. The SOLVD Investigators. *N Engl J Med* 1991;325:293-302.

Effect of metoprolol CR/XL in chronic heart failure: Metoprolol CR/XL Randomized Intervention Trial in Congestive Heart Failure (MERIT-HF). *Lancet* 1999;353:2001-2007.

Effects on enalapril on mortality in severe congestive heart failure: Results of the cooperative North Scandinavian Enalapril Survival Study (CONSENSUS). The CONSENSUS Trial Study Group. *N Engl J Med* 1987;316:1429-1435.

Eichhorn E, Bristow M: Medical therapy can improve the biological properties of the chronically failing heart: a new era in the treatment of heart failure. *Circulation* 1996;94:2285-2296.

Flather MD, Yusuf S, Kober L, et al: Long-term ACE-inhibitor therapy in patients with heart failure or left-ventricular dysfunction: a systematic overview of data from individual patients. *Lancet* 2000;355:1575-1581.

Franzosi MG, Santoro E, Zuanetti G, et al: Indications for ACE inhibitors in the early treatment of acute myocardial infarction: systematic overview of individual data from 100,000 patients in randomized trials. *Circulation* 1998;97:2202-2212.

Gogia H, Mehra A, Parikh S, et al: Prevention of tolerance to hemodynamic effects of nitrates with concomitant use of hydralazine in patients with chronic heart failure. *J Am Coll Cardiol* 1995;26:1575-1580.

Greenberg B, Quinones MA, Koilpillai C, et al: Effects of long-term enalapril therapy on cardiac structure and function in patients with left ventricular dysfunction: results of the SOLVD echocardiography study. *Circulation* 1995;91:2573-2581.

Hauptmann PJ, Kelly RA: Digitalis. *Circulation* 1999;99:1265-1270.

Heart Failure Society of America (HFSA) practice guidelines. HFSA guidelines for management of patients with heart failure caused by left ventricular systolic dysfunction—pharmacological approaches. *J Card Fail* 1999;5:357-382.

Ho KK, Anderson KM, Kannel WB, et al: Survival after the onset of congestive heart failure in Framingham Heart Study subjects. *Circulation* 1993;88:107-115.

Latini R, Maggioni AP, Flather M, et al: ACE inhibitor use in patients with myocardial infarction: summary of evidence from clinical trials. *Circulation* 1995;92:3132-3137.

Monane M, Bohn RL, Gurwitz JH, et al: Noncompliance with congestive heart failure therapy in the elderly. *Arch Intern Med* 1994; 154:433-437.

Packer M, Bristow MR, Cohn JN, et al: The effect of carvedilol on morbidity and mortality in patients with chronic heart failure. US Carvedilol Heart Failure Study Group. *N Engl J Med* 1996;334:1349-1355.

Packer M, Coats AJ, Fowler MB, et al: Effect of carvedilol on survival in severe chronic heart failure. *N Engl J Med* 2001;344:1651-1658.

Packer M, Gheorghiade M, Young JB, et al: Withdrawal of digoxin from patients with chronic heart failure treated with angiotensin-converting-enzyme inhibitors. RADIANCE Study. *N Engl J Med* 1993;329:1-7.

Pfeffer MA, Braunwald E, Moyé LA, et al: Effect of captopril on mortality and morbidity in patients with left ventricular dysfunction after myocardial infarction. Results of the survival and ventricular enlargement trial. The SAVE Investigators. *N Engl J Med* 1992;327:669-677.

Pitt B, Poole-Wilson PA, Segal R, et al: Effect of losartan compared with captopril on mortality in patients with symptomatic heart failure: randomized trial—the Losartan Heart Failure Survival Study ELITE II. *Lancet* 2000;355:1582-1587.

Pitt B, Zannad F, Remme WJ, et al: The effect of spironolactone on morbidity and mortality in patients with severe heart failure. Randomized Aldactone Evaluation Study Investigators. *N Engl J Med* 1999;341:709-717.

Sharpe N, Murphy J, Smith H, et al: Treatment of patients with symptomless left ventricular dysfunction after myocardial infarction. *Lancet* 1988;1:255-259.

Vinson JM, Rich MW, Sperry JC, et al: Early readmission of elderly patients with congestive heart failure. *J Am Geriatr Soc* 1990;38:1290-1295.

Young JB, Gheorghiade M, Uretsky BF, et al: Superiority of 'triple' drug therapy in heart failure: insights from the PROVED and RADIANCE trials. Prospective Randomized Study of Ventricular

Function and Efficacy of Digoxin. Randomized Assessment of Digoxin and Inhibitors of Angiotensin-Converting Enzyme. *J Am Coll Cardiol* 1998;32:686-692.

Yusuf S, Sleight P, Pogue J, et al: Effects of an angiotensin-converting-enzyme inhibitor, ramipril, on cardiovascular events in high-risk patients. The Heart Outcomes Prevention Evaluation Study Investigators. *N Engl J Med* 2000;342:145-153.

Index

282

S

T

tachyarrhythmias 207, 223, 246
tachycardia 42, 43, 49, 64, 81, 82, 215, 217, 223, 245
tachyphylaxis 64, 215
tachypnea 42, 210
Tegretol® 39
telemetry monitoring 212
tezosentan 234, 236
thalassemia 41
thrombocytopenia 217
thyroid disease 37, 50, 208
thyroid-stimulating hormone (TSH) 47
tissue inhibitors of metalloproteinases 21
titin 9, 11
tobacco 188, 195, 265
Toprol-XL® 124, 148, 150, 154, 162, 167
torsemide (Demadex®) 70, 256
toxemia 207
toxicity 38, 39, 64-66, 69, 215, 221, 223
Tracleer™ 234
trandolapril (Mavik®) 116
transforming growth factor-β (TGF-β) 96
trastuzumab (Herceptin®) 245
travel limitations 193
treatment algorithm 232

triamterene (Dyazide®, Maxzide®) 72
tricyclic antidepressants (TCAs) 192
tropomyosin 233
troponin C 230, 233
troponin T 9, 10
tubulin 9
tumor necrosis factor (TNF) 21
    TNF-α 19, 40, 51, 181

U

University Healthcare Consortium (UHC) 237, 239
US Carvedilol Trials program 148, 150-152, 157

V

valsartan (Diovan®) 122, 124, 126-128
Valsartan in Heart Failure Trial (Val-HeFT) 122, 124, 126-129, 258
valvular heart disease 33, 181, 186, 245, 264
Vaseretic® 72, 79
vasoconstriction 12, 96, 99, 106, 142, 161, 209, 222
vasodilation 76, 81, 84

NOTES